Ketogenic Recipes for Beginners

The revolutionary diet

for Women Over 50

Shannon Wood

TABLE OF CONTENTS

content within this book has been derived from various sources. Please consult a licensed professional before attempting any techniques outlined in this book. By reading this document, the reader agrees that under no circumstances is the author responsible for any losses, 5 direct or indirect, which are incurred as a result of the use of information contained within this document, including, but not limited to, — errors, omissions, or inaccuracies.

BREAKFAST

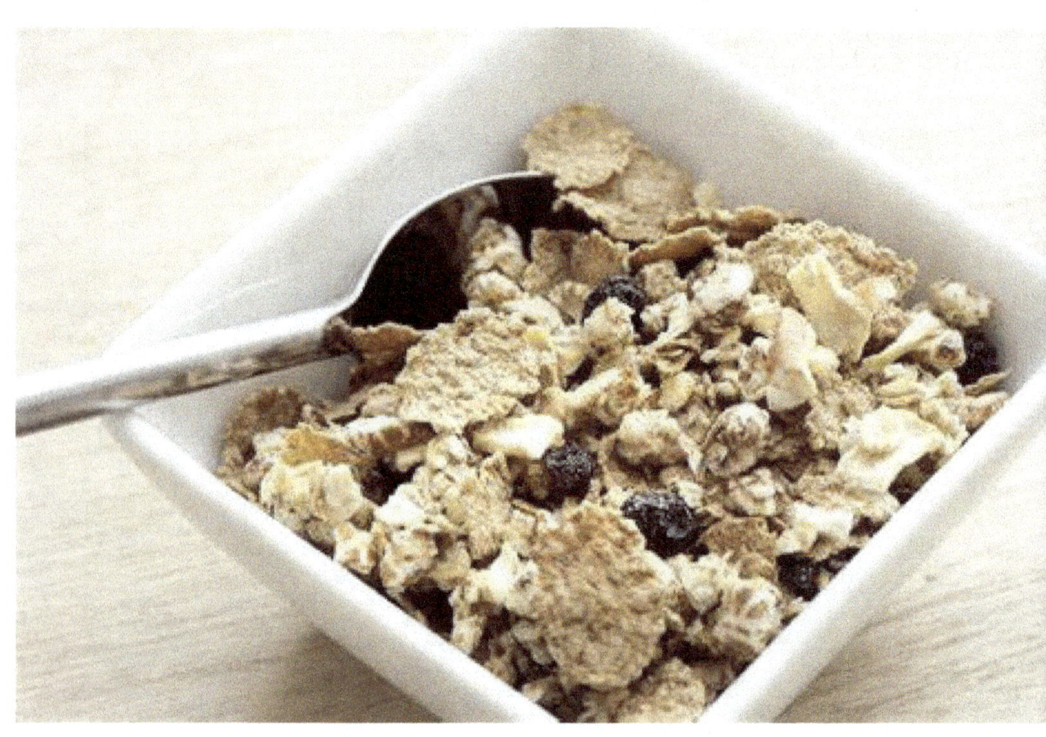

Breakfast Meatloaf

Servings: 4

Cooking Time: 35 minutes

Ingredients

- 1 teaspoon ghee
- 1 small yellow onion, chopped
- 1 pound sweet sausage, chopped
- 6 eggs
- 1 cup cheddar cheese, shredded
- 4 ounces cream cheese, soft
- Salt and black pepper to the taste
- 2 tablespoons scallions, chopped

Directions:

1. Mix eggs with salt, pepper, onion, sausage and half of the cream and whisk well.

2. Grease a meatloaf with the ghee, pour sausage and eggs mix, introduce in the oven at 350 degrees F and bake for minutes.

3. Take the meatloaf out of the oven, leave aside for a couple of minutes, spread the rest of the cream cheese on top and sprinkle scallions and cheddar cheese all over.

4. Introduce meatloaf in the oven again and bake for 5 minutes more.

5. After the time has passed, broil meatloaf for 3 minutes, leave it aside to cool down a bit, slice and serve it.

6. Enjoy!

Nutrition Info:

Calories 560, fat 32, fiber 1, carbs 6, protein 45

Coconut Muesli

Servings: 15

Preparation Time: 1 minute

Cooking Time: 8 minutes

Ingredients:

- Flaked coconut -unsweetened: 1 cup
- Sunflower seeds: 1 cup
- Pumpkin seeds: 1 cup
- Almonds -sliced: 1 cup
- Pecans: ½ cup
- Hemp hearts: ½ cup
- Cinnamon: 2 teaspoons
- Vanilla extract: ½ teaspoon
- Vanilla stevia: ¼ teaspoon

Directions:

1. Toss together all the ingredients in a baking pan.
2. Bake for 7-8 minutes at 350 degrees Fahrenheit.
3. Leave to cool.
4. Serve with almond milk.

Nutrition Value:

200 Cal, 17.8 g total fat, 3 mg sodium, 6.1 g carb., 3.3g fiber, 6.9 g protein.

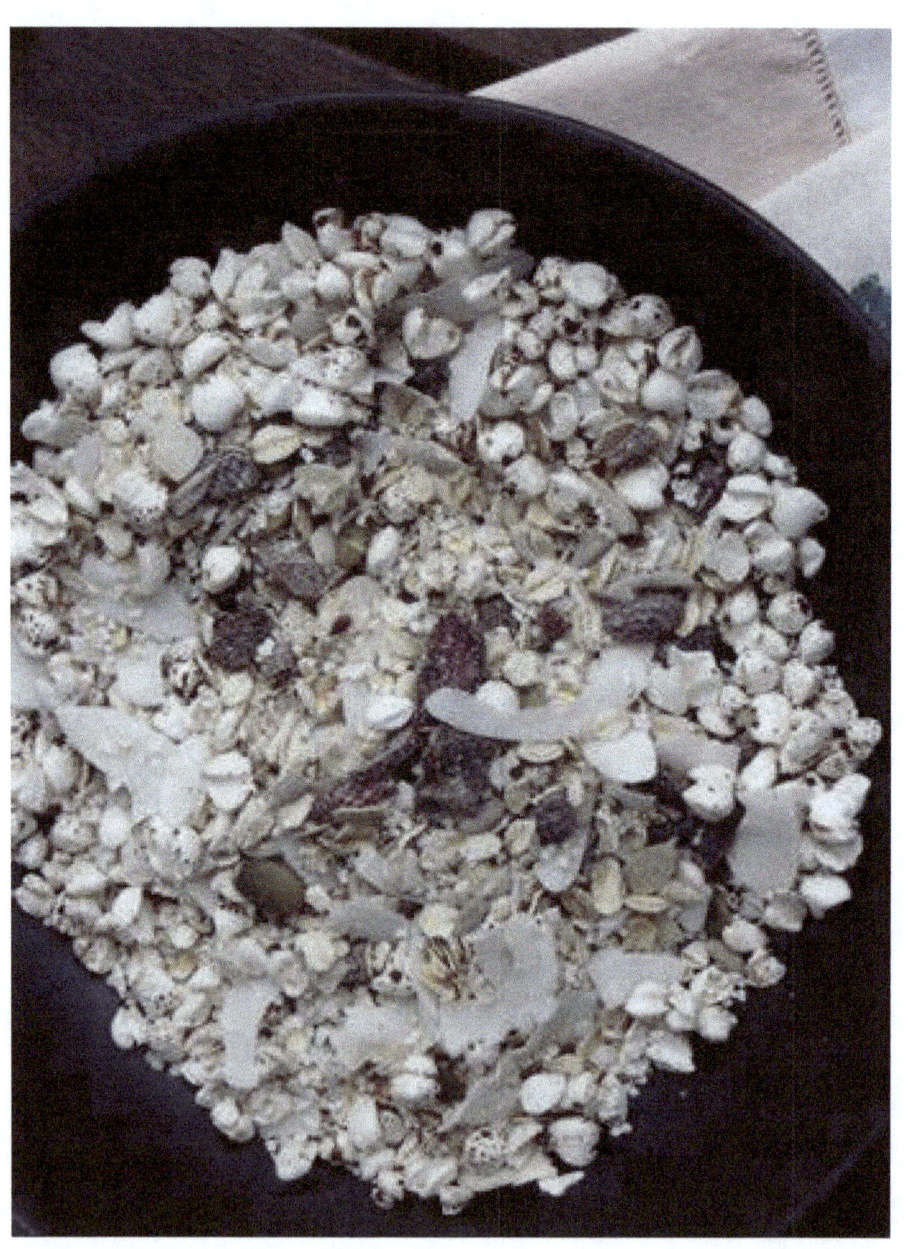

Fruit & Nut Cereal

Servings: 1

Preparation Time: 5 minutes

Ingredients:

- Strawberries -chopped: 2
- Blueberries: 2 tablespoon
- Almonds -chopped: 3 tablespoon
- Walnuts -chopped: 2 tablespoon
- Pecans -chopped: 3 tablespoon
- Sweetener: 3 tablespoon
- Coconut milk: for serving

Directions:

1. Combine together all the ingredients in a bowl except the coconut milk.

2. Stir in the coconut milk.

Nutrition Value:

308 Cal, 32.59 g total fat, 2.96g carb., 5.79g fiber, 7.88 g protein.

Blueberry Porridge

Servings: 2

Preparation Time: 5 minutes

Cooking Time: 5 minutes

Ingredients:

- Almond milk: 1 cup
- Ground flaxseed: ¼ cup
- Coconut flour: ¼ cup
- Cinnamon: 1 teaspoon
- Vanilla extract: 1 teaspoon
- Liquid stevia: 10 drops
- Salt: a pinch

Directions:

1. Heat the almond milk over a low flame and whisk in the flour, flaxseed, salt, and cinnamon.
2. Mix in the vanilla extract and stevia once it begins to bubble.
3. Remove from the flame once the mixture is thick.
4. Serve topped with shaved coconut, pumpkin seeds, and some blueberries.

Nutrition Value:

405 Cal, 34 g total fat, 8 g net carb., 10 g protein.

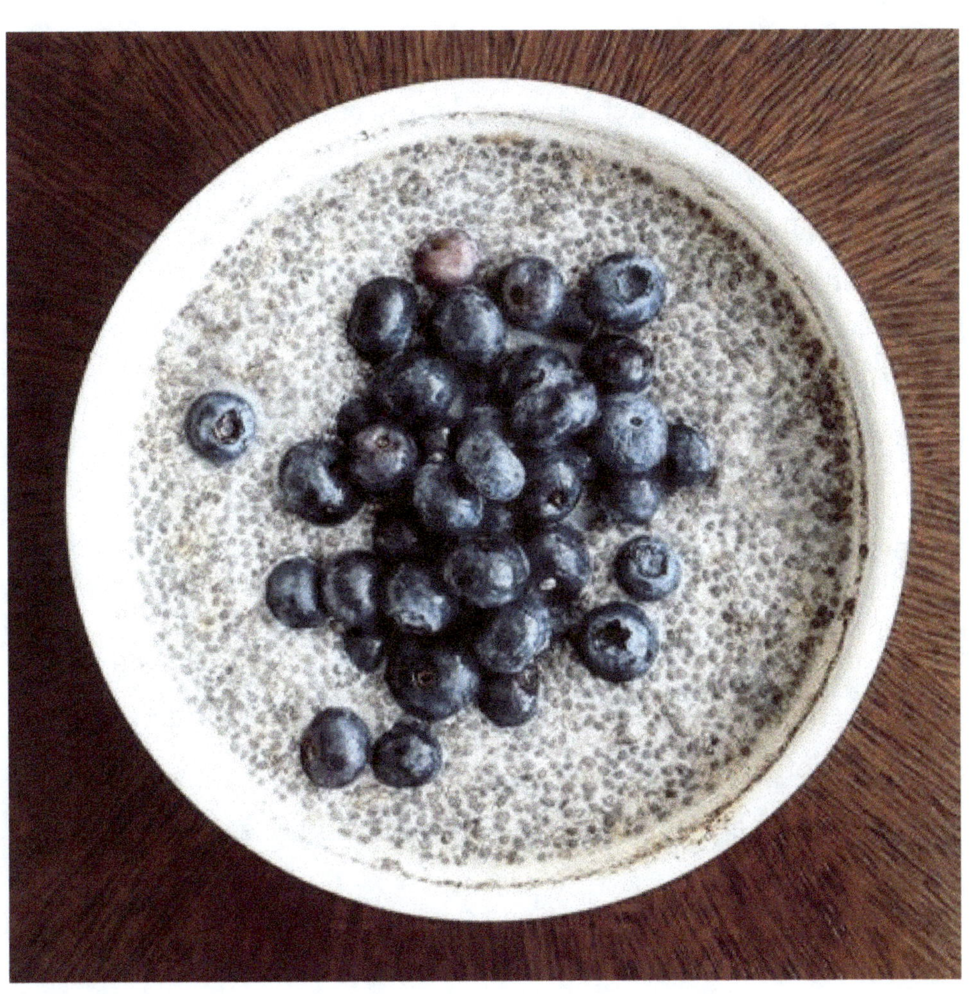

Morning Berry-green Smoothie

Servings: 4

Cooking Time: 5 minutes

Ingredients

- 1 avocado, pitted and sliced
- 3 cups mixed blueberries and strawberries
- 2 cups unsweetened almond milk
- 6 tbsp heavy cream
- 2 tbsp erythritol
- 1 cup of ice cubes
- ⅓ cup nuts and seeds mix

Directions:

1. Combine the avocado slices, blueberries, strawberries, almond milk, heavy cream, erythritol, ice cubes, nuts and seeds in a smoothie maker; blend at high speed until smooth and uniform.

2. Pour the smoothie into drinking glasses and serve immediately.

Nutrition Info (Per Serving): Kcal 360, Fat 33.3g, Net Carbs 6g, Protein 6g

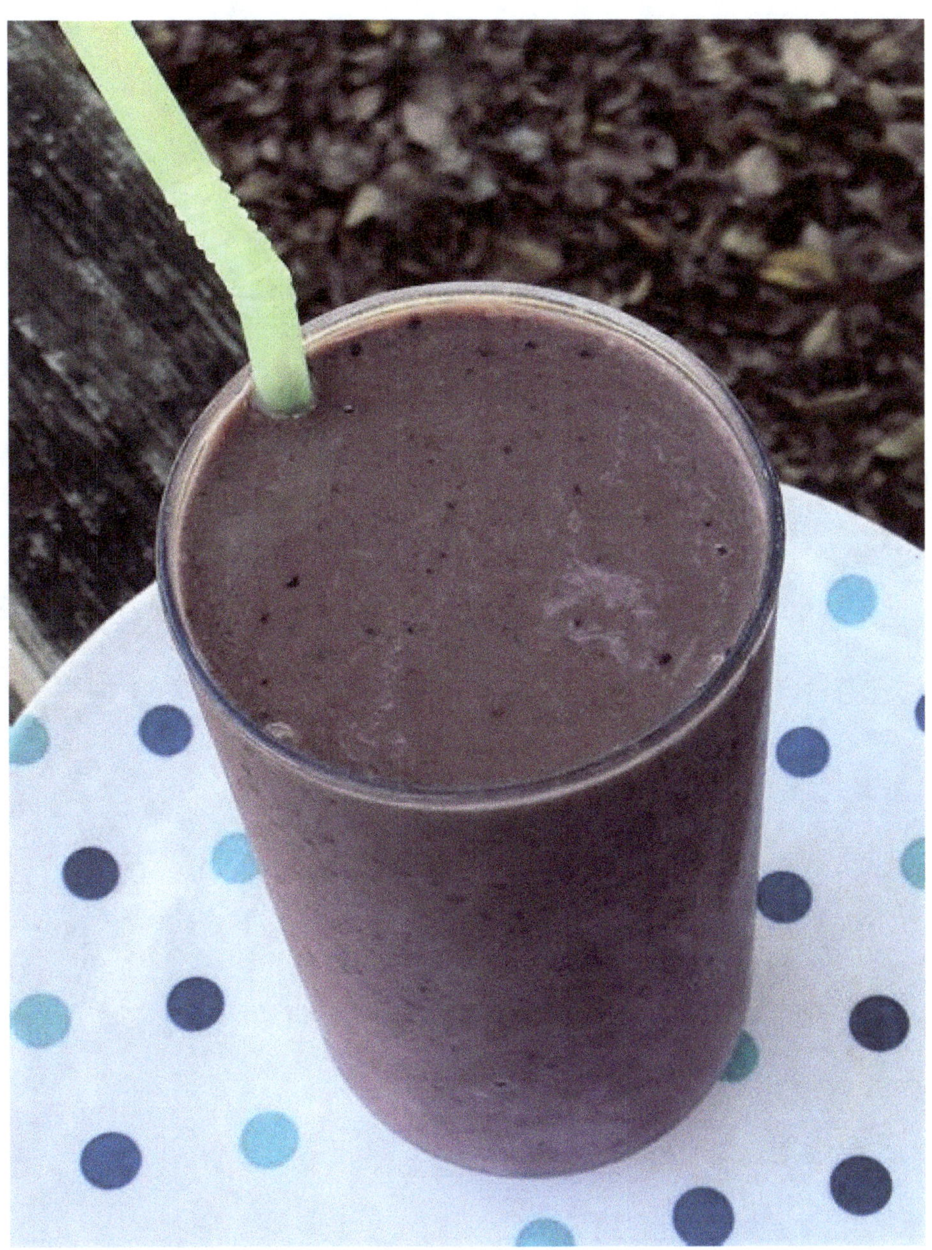

BRUNCH

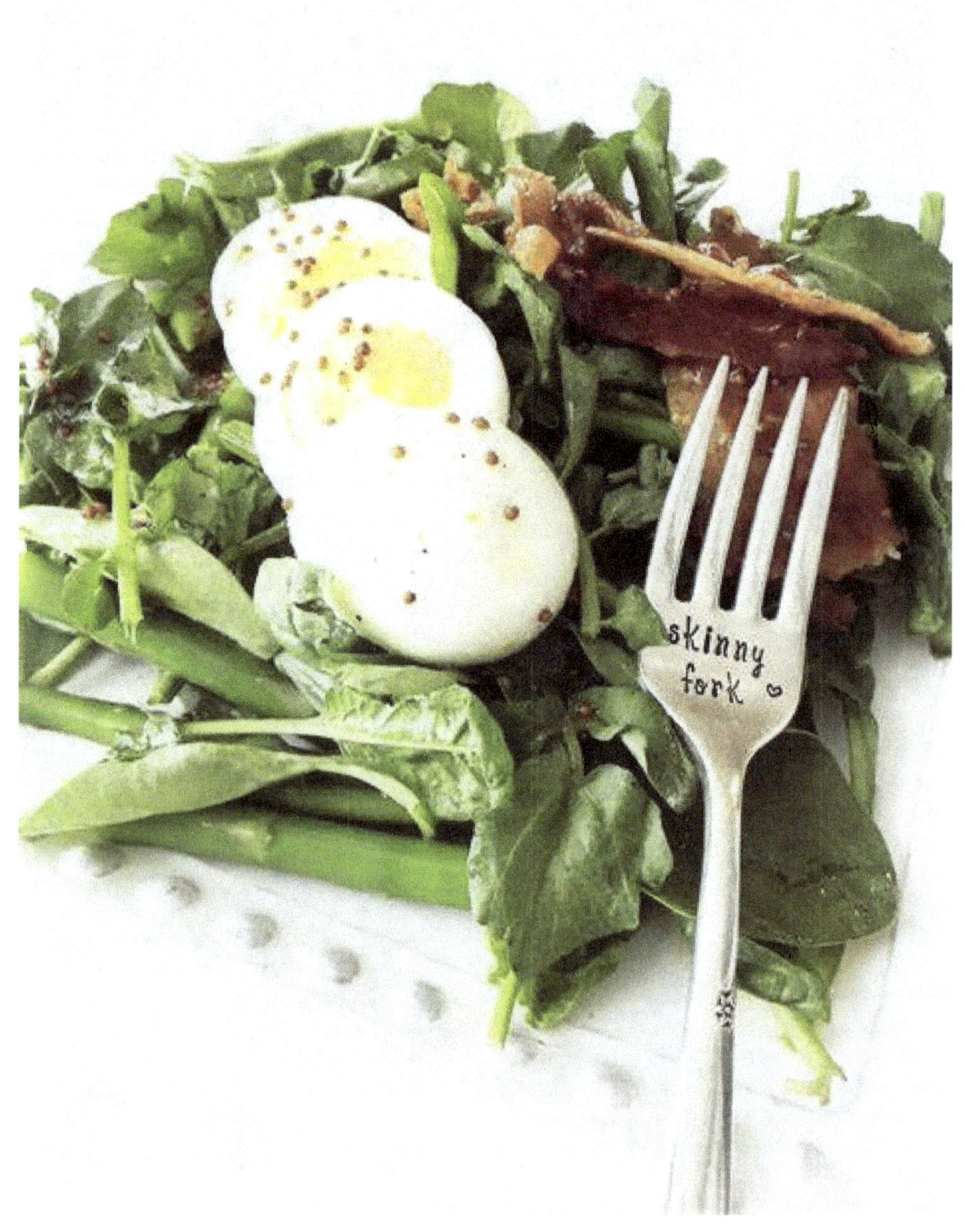

Avocado Halloumi Scones

Servings: 4

Cooking Time: 35 minutes

Ingredients

- 1 cup crumbled halloumi cheese
- 2 cups almond flour
- 3 tsp baking powder
- ½ cup butter, cold
- 1 avocado, pitted and mashed
- 1 large egg
- 1/3 cup buttermilk

Directions:

1. Preheat oven to 350° F; then line a baking sheet with parchment paper. In a bowl, combine flour and baking powder.

2. Add butter and mix. Top with halloumi cheese, avocado, and combine again.

3. Whisk the egg with the buttermilk and stir in the halloumi mix. Mold 8- scones out to the batter.

4. Place on the baking sheet, then bakes for 25 minutes or until the scones turn a golden color.

5. Let cool.

Nutrition Info (Per Serving): Cal 432; Net Carbs 2.3g; Fat 42g; Protein 10g

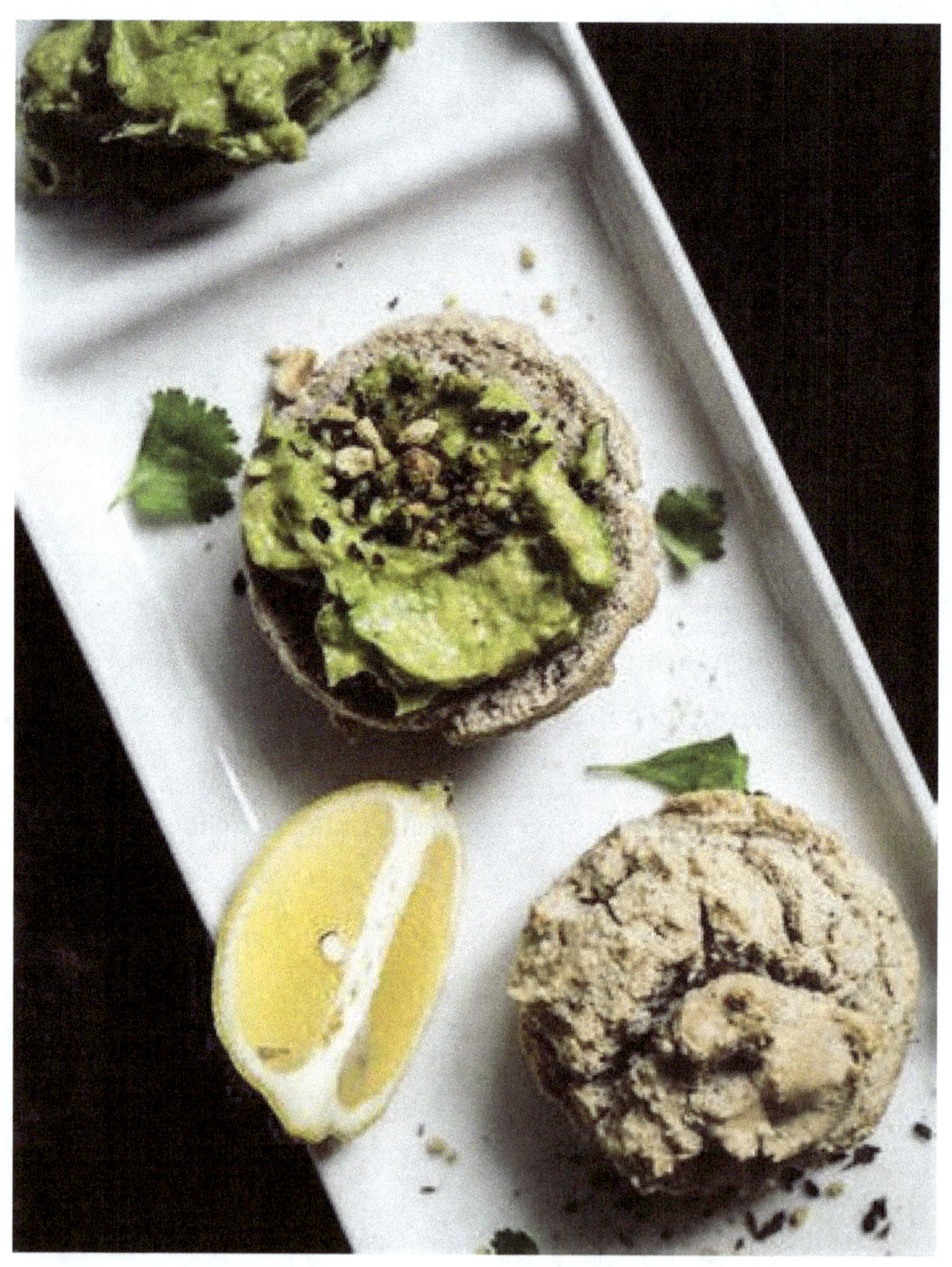

Lunch Spinach Rolls

Servings: 16

Cooking Time: 15 minutes

Ingredients

- 6 tablespoons coconut flour
- ½ cup almond flour
- 2 and ½ cups mozzarella cheese, shredded
- 2 eggs
- A pinch of salt

For the filling:

- 4 ounces cream cheese
- 6 ounces spinach, torn
- A drizzle of avocado oil
- A pinch of salt
- ¼ cup parmesan, grated
- Mayonnaise for serving

Directions:

1. Heat up a pan. Oil over medium heat, add some spinach and cook for 2 minutes.
2. Add parmesan, a pinch of salt and cream cheese, stir well, take off the heat and leave aside for now.

3. Put mozzarella cheese in a heatproof bowl and microwave for seconds.

4. Add eggs, salt, coconut and almond flour and stir everything.

5. Place dough on a lined cutting board, place parchment paper on top and flatten dough with a rolling pin.

6. Divide dough into 1rectangles, spread spinach mix on each and roll them into cigar shapes.

7. Place all rolls on a lined baking sheet, introduce in the oven at 350 degrees F and bake for 15 minutes.

8. Leave rolls to cool down for a few minutes before serving them with some mayo on top.

9. Enjoy!

Nutrition Info: calories 500, fat 65, fiber 4, carbs 14, protein 32

Herbed Coconut Flour Bread

Servings: 2

Cooking Time: 3 minutes

Ingredients

- 4 tbsp coconut flour
- ½ tsp baking powder
- ½ tsp dried thyme
- 2 tbsp whipping cream
- 2 eggs

Seasoning:

- ½ tsp oregano
- 2 tbsp avocado oil

Directions:

1. Take a medium bowl, place all the ingredients in it and then whisk until incorporated and smooth batter comes together.

2. Distribute the mixture evenly between two mugs and then microwave for a minute and 30 seconds until cooked. When done, take out bread from the mugs, cut it into slices, and then serve.

Nutrition Info:

309 Calories; 26.1 g Fats; 9.3 g Protein; 4.3 g Net Carb; 5 g Fiber

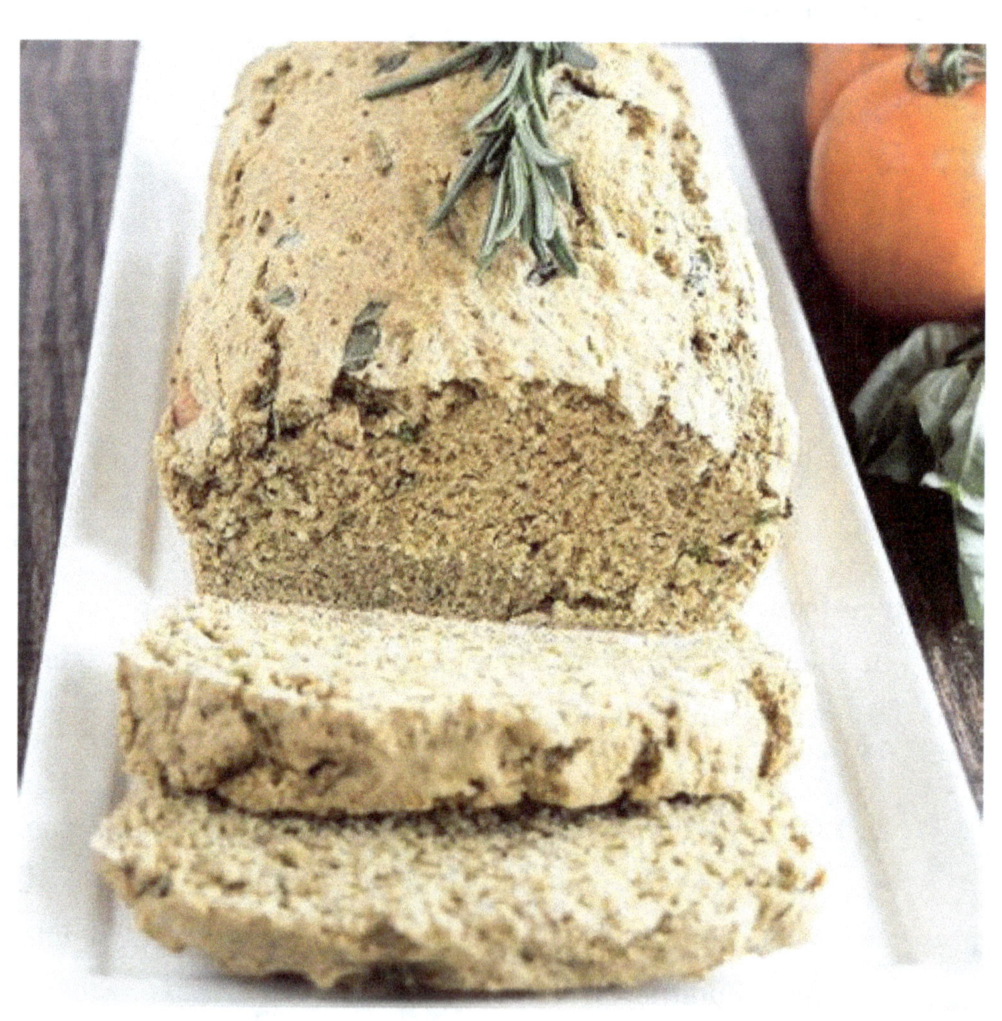

Simple Asparagus Lunch

Servings: 4

Cooking Time: 10 minutes

Ingredients

- 2 egg yolks
- Salt and black pepper to the taste
- ¼ cup ghee
- 1 tablespoon lemon juice
- A pinch of cayenne pepper
- 40 asparagus spears

Directions:

1. In a bowl, whisk egg yolks very well.
2. Transfer this to a small pan over low heat.
3. Add lemon juice and whisk well.
4. Add ghee and whisk until it melts.
5. Add salt, pepper, cayenne pepper and whisk again well.
6. Heat up a pan at medium-high heat, add asparagus spears and fry them for 5 minutes.
7. Divide asparagus between plates, drizzle the sauce you've made on top and serve.
8. Enjoy!

Nutrition Info: calories 150, fat 13, fiber 6, carbs 2, protein 3

Herbed Keto Bread

Servings: 6

Cooking Time: 40 minutes

Ingredients

- 5 eggs
- ½ tsp cream of tartar
- 2 cups almond flour
- 3 tablespoons butter, melted
- 3 tsp baking powder
- 1 tsp salt
- 1 tsp dried rosemary
- ½ tsp dried oregano
- 1 tbsp sunflower seeds
- 2 tbsp sesame seeds

Directions:

1. Preheat oven to 360° F, then grease a loaf pan with cooking spray. Combine the eggs with cream of tartar until the formation of stiff peaks happens. In a food processor, place in the baking powder, flour, salt, and butter and blitz to incorporate fully.

2. Stir in the egg mixture. Ladle the batter into the prepared loaf pan. Spread the loaf with sesame seeds, dried rosemary, sunflower seeds, and oregano and bake for 35 minutes. Serve with butter.

Nutrition Info (Per Serving): Kcal 115, Fat: 10.2g, Net Carbs: 1g, Protein: 3.9g

SOUP AND STEWS

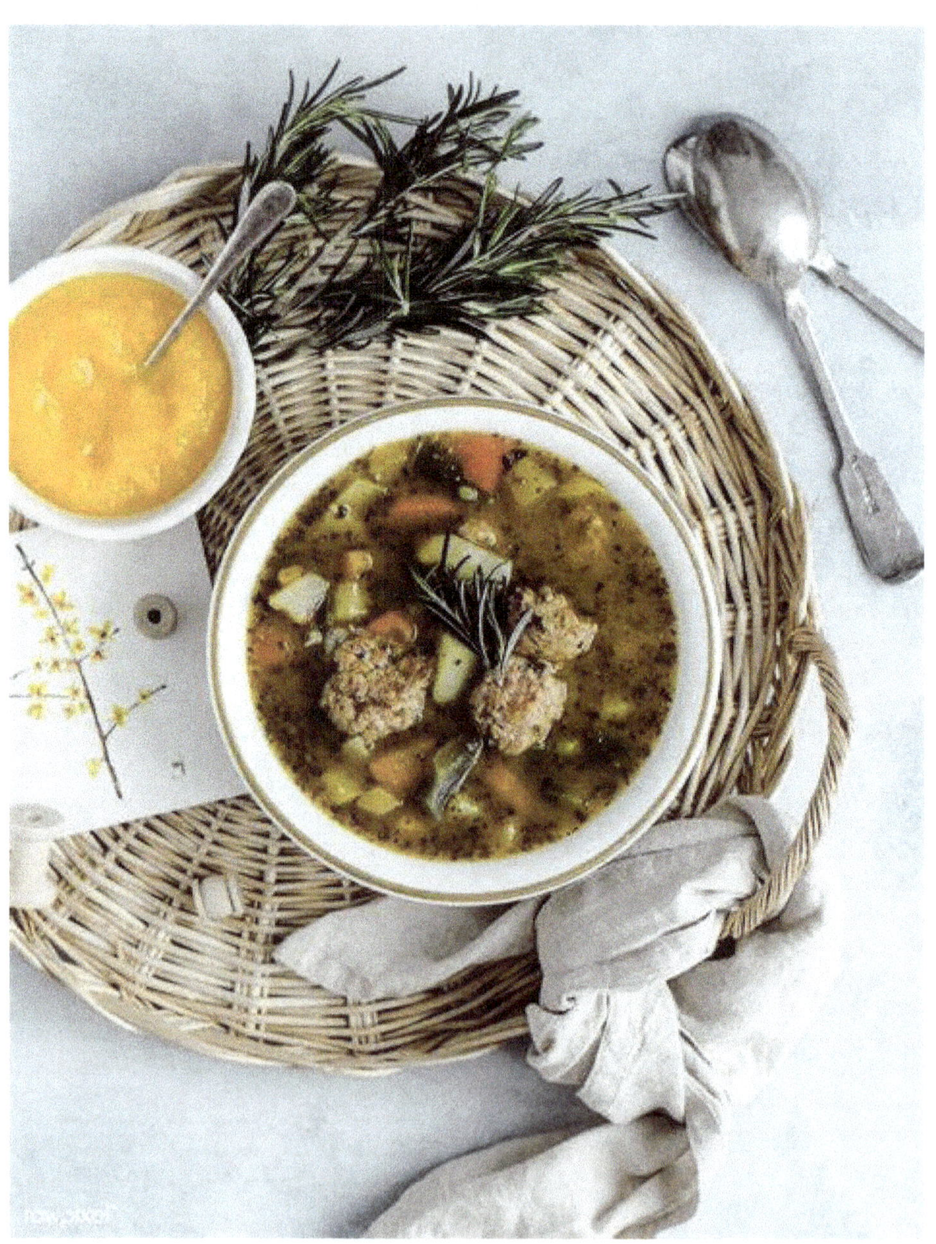

Mixed Mushroom Soup

Servings: 4

Cooking Time: 35 minutes

Ingredients

- 5 oz white button mushrooms, chopped
- 5 oz cremini mushrooms, chopped
- 5 oz shiitake mushrooms, chopped
- 4 oz unsalted butter
- 1 small onion, finely chopped
- 1 clove garlic, minced
- ½ lb celery root, chopped
- ½ tsp dried rosemary
- 4 cups of water
- 1 vegan stock cube, crushed
- 1 tbsp plain vinegar
- 1 cup coconut cream
- 6 leaves basil, chopped

Directions:

1. Melt butter in a saucepan. Sauté onion, garlic, mushrooms, and celery root until golden brown and fragrant, about 6 minutes.

2. Reserve some mushrooms for garnishing. Add in rosemary, water, stock cube, and vinegar.

3. Stir and bring to a boil for 6 minutes.

4. Reduce the heat and simmer for minutes.

5. Mix in coconut cream and puree.

6. Spoon into bowls garnished with the reserved mushrooms
   and basil.

Nutrition Info (Per Serving): Cal 506; Fat 46g; Net Carbs 12g; Protein 8g

Creamy Cauliflower Soup with Bacon Chips

Servings: 4

Cooking Time: 25 minutes

Ingredients

- 2 tbsp ghee
- 1 onion, chopped
- 2 head cauliflower, cut into florets
- 2 cups of water
- Salt and black pepper to taste
- 3 cups almond milk
- 1 cup shredded white cheddar cheese
- 3 bacon strips

Directions:

1. Melt the ghee into a saucepan, over medium heat and sauté the onion for 3 minutes until fragrant.

2. Include the cauli florets, sauté for 3 minutes to slightly soften, add the water, and season with salt and black pepper. Bring to a boil; then, you need to reduce the heat to low. Cover and cook for 10 minutes. Puree cauliflower with an immersion blender until the ingredients are evenly combined, and stir in the almond milk and cheese until the cheese melts. Adjust taste with salt and black pepper.

3. In a non-stick skillet over high heat, fry the bacon until crispy. Divide soup between serving bowls, top with crispy bacon, and serve hot.

Nutrition Info (Per Serving): Kcal 402, Fat 37g, Net Carbs 6g, Protein 8g

Roasted Tomato Cream

Servings: 8

Cooking Time: 1 Hour

Ingredients

- 1 jalapeno pepper, chopped
- 4 garlic cloves, minced
- 2 pounds cherry tomatoes, cut in halves
- 1 yellow onion, cut into wedges
- Salt and black pepper to the taste
- ¼ cup olive oil
- ½ teaspoon oregano, dried
- 4 cups chicken stock
- ¼ cup basil, chopped
- ½ cup parmesan, grated

Directions:

1. Spread tomatoes and onion in a baking dish. Add garlic and chili pepper, season with salt, pepper and oregano and drizzle the oil.
2. Toss to coat and bake in the oven at 4 degrees F for 30 minutes.
3. Take tomatoes to mix out of the oven, transfer to a pot, add stock and heat everything up over medium-high heat.

4. Bring to a boil, cover the pot, reduce heat and simmer for 20 minutes.

5. Blend using an immersion blender, add salt and pepper to the taste and basil, stir and ladle into soup bowls.

6. Sprinkle parmesan on top and serve.

7. Enjoy!

Nutrition Info: calories 140, fat 2, fiber 2, carbs 5, protein 8

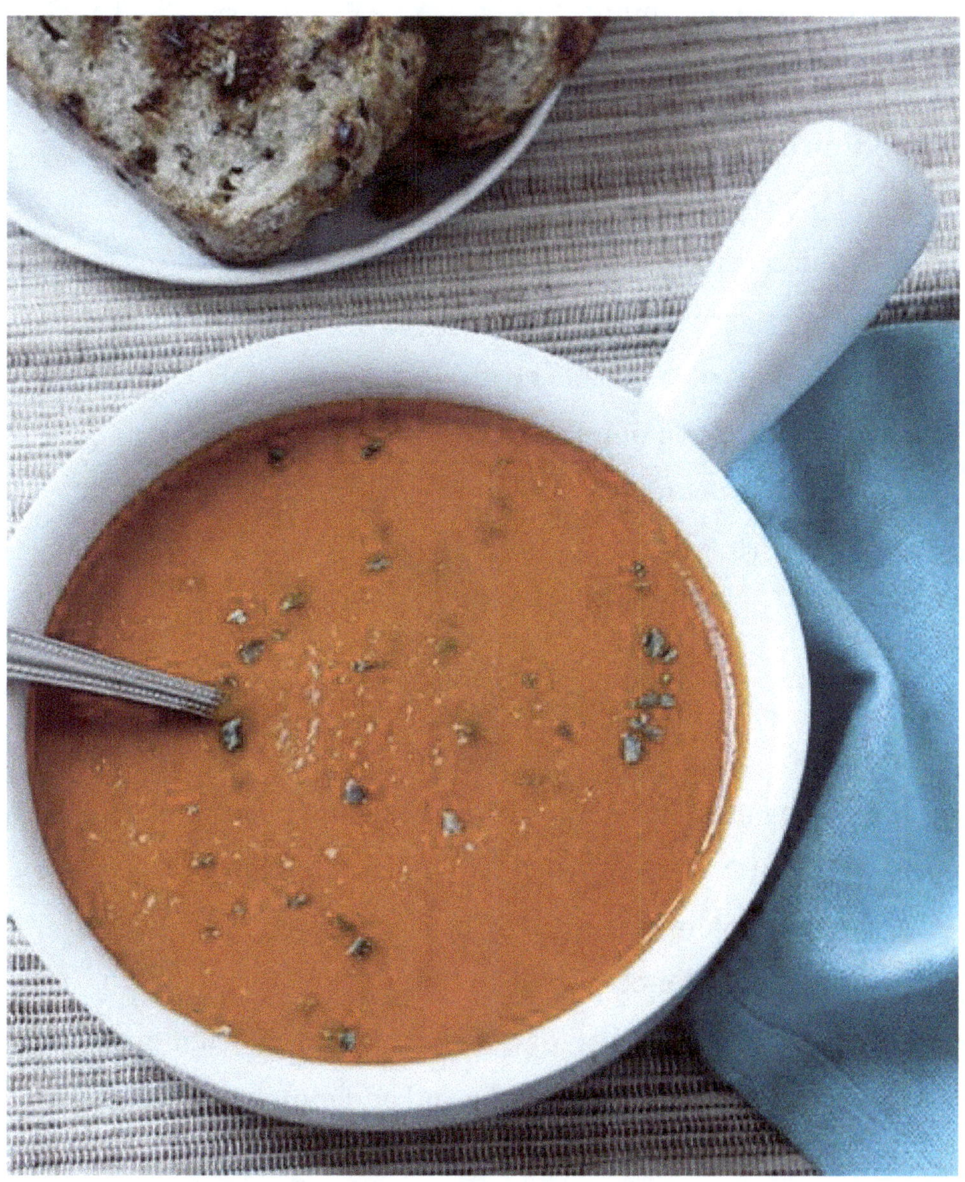

Nutmeg Pumpkin Soup

Preparation Time: 15 minutes

Cooking Time: 20 minutes

Servings: 4

Ingredients:

- 1 tablespoon of butter
- 1 onion (diced)
- 1 16-ounce can of pumpkin puree
- 1 1/3 cups of vegetable broth
- 1/2 tablespoon of nutmeg
- 1/2 tablespoon of sugar Salt (to taste)
- Pepper (to taste)
- 3 cups of soymilk or any milk as a substitute

Directions:

1. Using a large saucepan, add onion to margarine and cook it between 3 and 5 minutes until the onion is clear
2. Add pumpkin puree, vegetable broth, sugar, pepper, and other ingredients and stir to combine.
3. Cook in medium heat for between 10 and fifteen minutes
4. Before serving the soup, taste and add more spices, pepper, and salt if necessary
5. Serve soup and enjoy it!

Nutrition:

Calories: 165 Fat: 4.9g Fiber: 11.9g Carbohydrates: 3.5 g Protein: 4.2g

Thai Coconut Vegetable Soup

Preparation Time: 15 minutes

Cooking Time: 20 minutes

Servings: 4

Ingredients:

- onion (diced)
- bell peppers (red, diced)
- 1/4 teaspoon of cayenne
- 1/2 tablespoon of coriander
- 1/2 tablespoon of cumin
- 4 tablespoons of olive oil
- 1 can of chickpeas
- 1 carrot (sliced)
- 3 cloves of garlic
- 1/2 cup of basil or cilantro (fresh chopped)
- 1 teaspoon of salt
- 3 limes (freshly squeezed juice)
- 1/2 cup of vegetable broth
- 1 cup of coconut milk
- 1 cup of peanut butter
- 21/2 cups of tomatoes (finely diced)

Directions:

1. Sauté garlic and onions. Make ingredients to be soft for at least 3 to 5 minutes

2. Leaving out basil, add the rest of the ingredients and allow it to simmer. Cook over low heat for an hour

3. Put the half amount to the food processor, allow it to be very smooth, and return to the pot

4. Add either basil or cilantro, and your coconut food is ready. Before serving the soup, taste and add more seasoning if necessary. Serve, and enjoy!

Nutrition:

Calories: 151 Fat: 6.9g Fiber: 12.5g Carbohydrates: 3.1 g Protein: 4.9g

MAIN

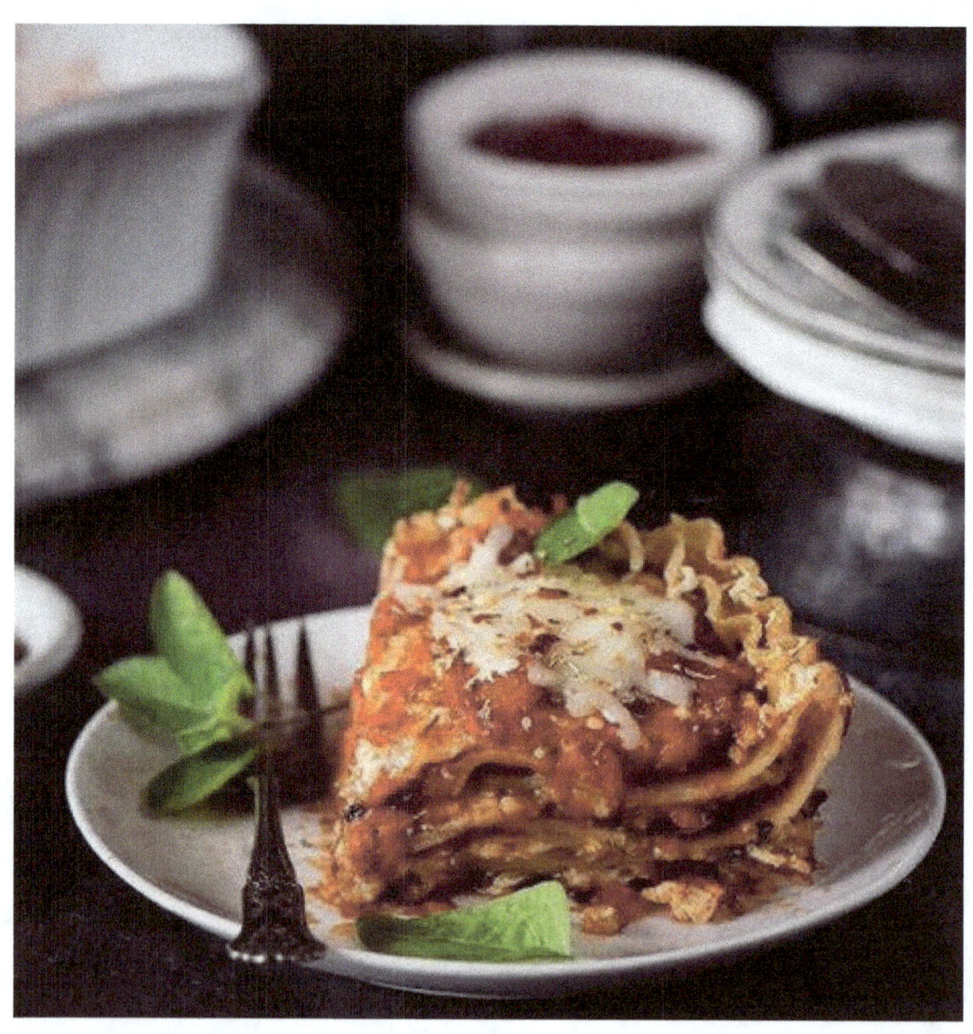

Cheesy Bacon Squash Spaghetti

Preparation Time: 30 minutes

Cooking Time: 50 minutes

Servings: 4

Ingredients:

- 2 pounds spaghetti squash
- 2 pounds bacon
- 1/2 cup of butter
- 2 cups of shredded parmesan cheese
- Salt
- Black pepper

Directions:

1. Let the oven preheat to 375° F.

2. Trim or remove each spaghetti squash stem, slice into rings no more than an inch wide, and take out the seeds.

3. Lay the sliced rings down on the baking sheet, bake for 40-45 minutes.

4. It is ready when the strands separate easily when a fork is used to scrape it. Let it cool.

5. Cook sliced up bacon until crispy. Take out and let it cool.

6. Take off the shell on each ring, separate each strand with a fork, and put them in a bowl.

7. Heat the strands in a microwave to get them warm, put in butter, and stir around until the butter melts.

8. Pour in parmesan cheese and bacon crumbles, and add salt and pepper to your taste.

9. Enjoy.

Nutrition:

Calories: 398 Fat: 12.5g Fiber: 9.4g Carbohydrates: 4.1 g Protein: 5.1g

Spinach and Zucchini Lasagna

Preparation Time: 15 minutes

Cooking Time: 30 minutes

Servings: 4

Ingredients:

- zucchinis, sliced
- Salt and black pepper to taste
- 2 cups ricotta cheese
- 2 cups shredded mozzarella cheese
- 3 cups tomato sauce
- 1 cup baby spinach

Directions:

1. Let the oven heat to 375 and grease a baking dish with cooking spray. Put the zucchini slices in a colander and sprinkle with salt.
2. Let sit and drain liquid for 5 minutes and pat dry with paper towels.
3. Mix the ricotta, mozzarella cheese, salt, and black pepper to evenly combine and spread 1/4 cup of the mixture in the bottom of the baking dish.
4. Layer 1/3 of the zucchini slices on top, spread 1 cup of tomato sauce over, and scatter a 1/3 cup of spinach on top. Repeat process.

5. Grease one end of foil with cooking spray and cover the baking dish with the foil.

6. Let it bake for about 35 minutes. And bake further for 5 to 10 minutes or until the cheese has a nice golden-brown color.

7. Remove the dish, sit for 5 minutes, make slices of the lasagna, and serve warm.

Nutrition:

Calories: 376 Fat: 14.1g Fiber: 11.3g Carbohydrates: 2.1 g Protein: 9.5g

Tomato Artichoke Pizza

Servings: 4

Cooking Time: 40 minutes

Ingredients

- 2 oz canned artichokes, cut into wedges
- 2 tbsp flax seed powder
- 4¼ oz grated broccoli
- 6¼ oz grated Parmesan
- ½ tsp salt
- 2 tbsp tomato sauce
- 2 oz mozzarella cheese, grated
- 1 garlic clove, thinly sliced
- 1 tbsp dried oregano
- Green olives for garnish

Directions:

1. Preheat oven to 350° F, then line a baking sheet with parchment paper.
2. In a bowl, mix flax seed powder and 6 tbsp water and allow thickening for 5 minutes.
3. When the flax egg is ready, add broccoli, 4 ½ ounces of Parmesan cheese, salt, and stir to combine.
4. Pour the mixture into the baking sheet and bake until the crust is lightly browned, 20 minutes. Remove from oven

and spread tomato sauce on top, sprinkle with the remaining Parmesan and mozzarella cheeses, add artichokes and garlic. Spread oregano on top.

5. Bake pizza for minutes at 420° F. Garnish with olives.

Nutrition Info (Per Serving): Cal 860; Net Carbs 10g; Fat 63g; Protein 55g

Cauliflower Risotto with Mushrooms

Servings: 4

Cooking Time: 15 minutes

Ingredients

- 2 shallots, diced
- 3 tbsp olive oil
- ¼ cup veggie broth
- ⅓ cup Parmesan cheese, shredded
- 2 tbsp butter
- 3 tbsp chopped chives
- 2 pounds mushrooms, sliced
- 4 cups cauliflower rice
- Salt and black pepper to taste
- 2 tbsp parsley, chopped

Directions:

1. Heat olive oil in a saucepan over medium heat. Add the mushrooms and shallots and cook for about 5 minutes until tender. Remove from the pan and set aside.

2. Add in the cauliflower, broth, salt, and black pepper, and cook until the liquid is absorbed about 4-5 minutes. Stir in butter and Parmesan cheese until the cheese is melted. Sprinkle with parsley to serve.

Nutrition Info (Per Serving):

Kcal 264, Fat: 18g, Net Carbs: 8.4g

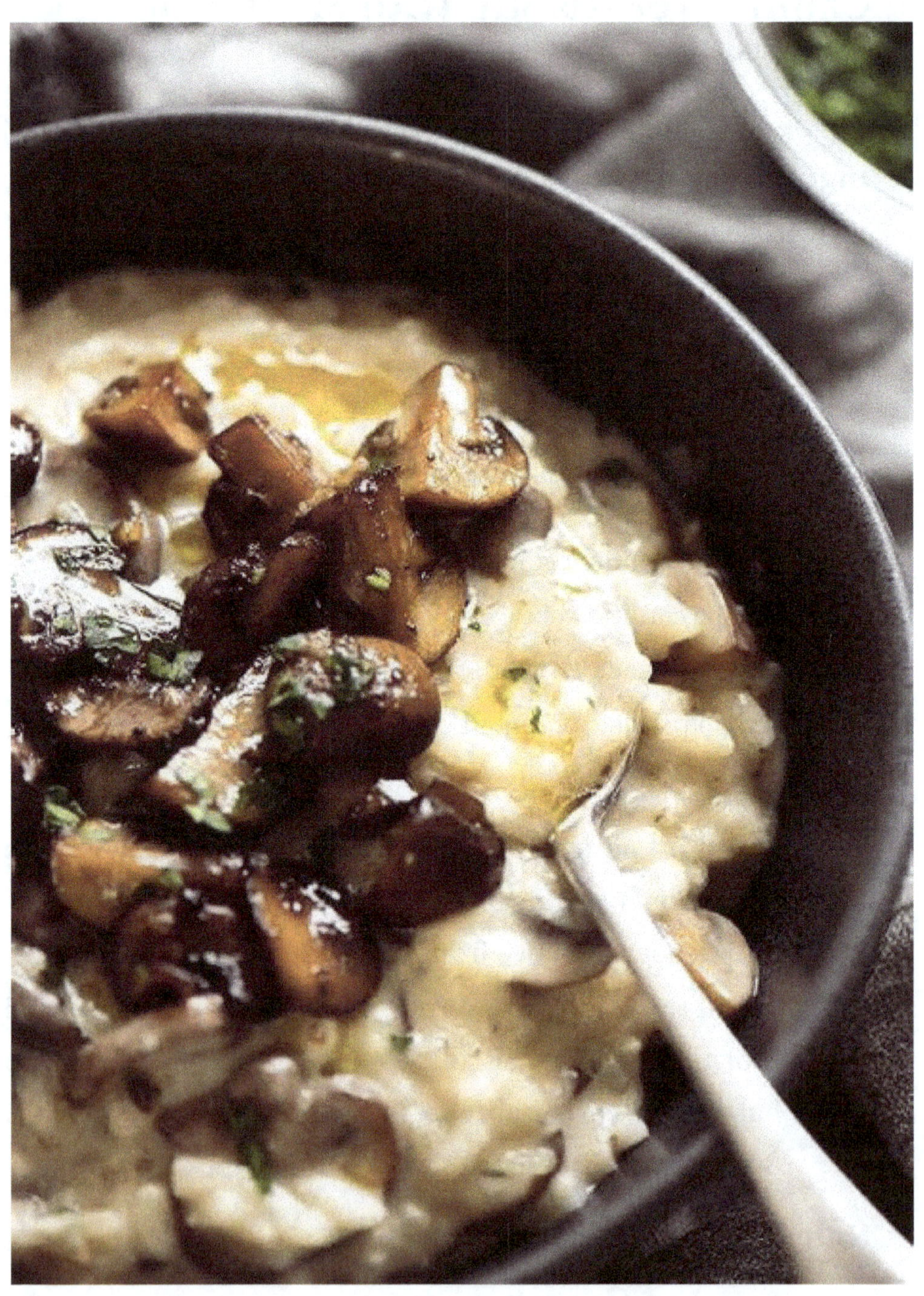

MEAT

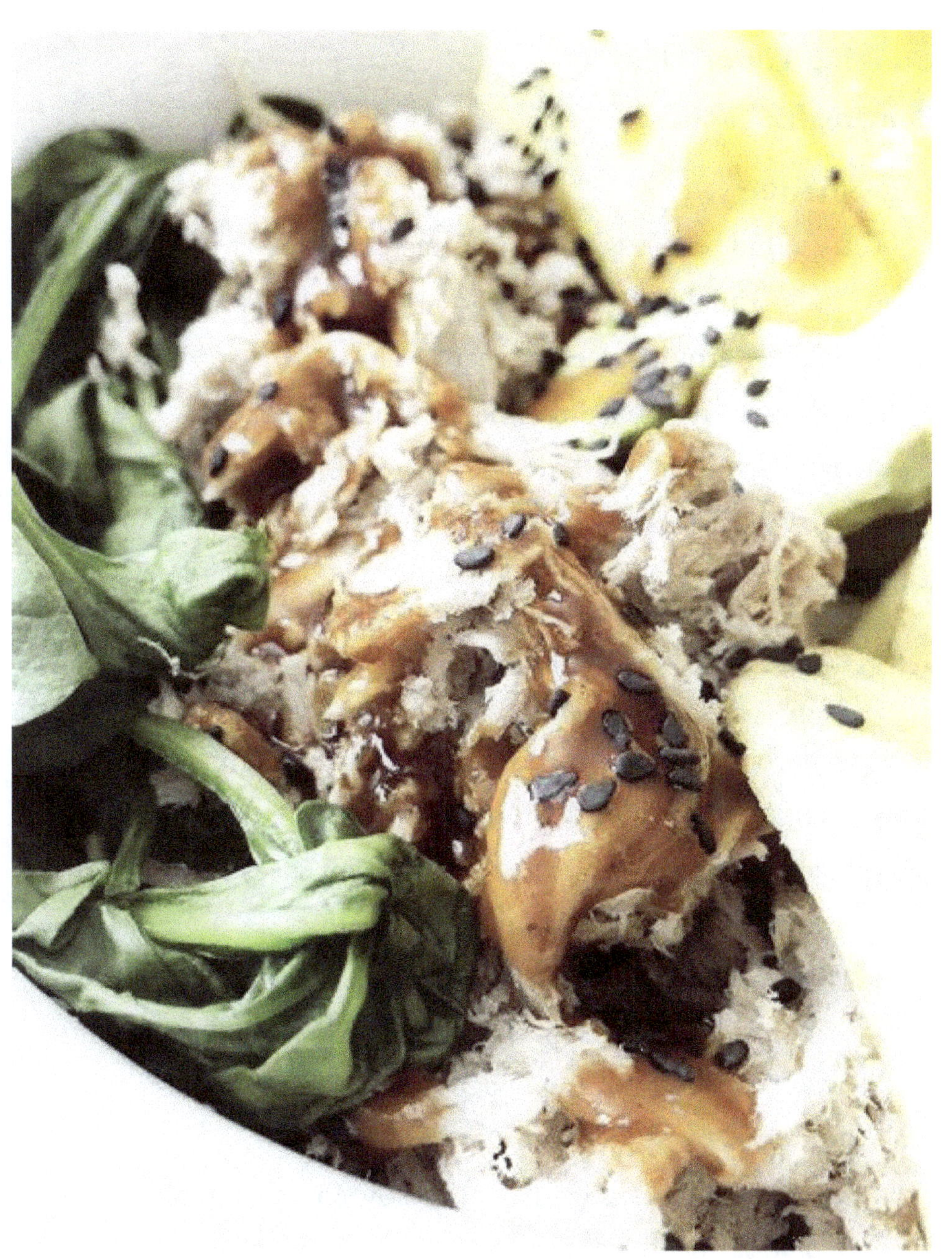

Kalua Pork with Cabbage

Preparation Time: 10 minutes

Cooking Time: 8 hrs.

Servings: 4

Ingredients:

- 1-pound boneless pork butt roast
- Pink Himalayan salt
- Freshly ground black pepper
- tablespoon smoked paprika or Liquid Smoke
- 1/2 cup of water
- 1/2 head cabbage, chopped

Directions:

1. With the crock insert in place, preheat the slow cooker to low.

2. Generously season the pork roast with pink Himalayan salt, pepper, and smoked paprika.

3. Place the pork roast in the slow-cooker insert, and add the water. Cover and cook on low for 7 hours.

4. Transfer the cooked pork roast to a plate. Put the chopped cabbage in the bottom of the slow cooker, and put the pork roast back in on the cabbage. Cover and cook the cabbage and pork roast for 1 hour.

5. Remove the pork roast from the slow cooker and place it on a baking sheet. Use two forks to shred the pork.

6. Serve the shredded pork hot with the cooked cabbage.

7. Reserve the liquid from the slow cooker to remoisten the pork and cabbage when reheating leftovers.

Nutrition:

Calories: 451 Fat: 19.3g Fiber: 11.2g Carbohydrates: 2.1 g Protein: 14.3g

Pork Chops in Blue Cheese Sauce

Preparation Time: 5 minutes

Cooking Time: 10 minutes

Servings: 2

Ingredients:

- boneless pork chops
- Pink Himalayan salt
- Freshly ground black pepper
- 2 tablespoons butter
- 1/3 cup blue cheese crumbles
- 1/3 cup heavy (whipping) cream
- 1/3 cup sour cream

Directions:

1. Dry the pork chops and season with pink Himalayan salt and pepper.
2. In a medium skillet over medium heat, melt the butter. When the butter melts and is very hot, add the pork chops and sear on each side for 3 minutes.
3. The pork chops must be transferred to a plate and let rest for 3 to 5 minutes.
4. In a preheated pan, melt the blue cheese crumbles, frequently stirring, so they don't burn.

5. Add the cream and the sour cream to the pan with the blue cheese. Let simmer for a few minutes, stirring occasionally.

6. For an extra kick of flavor in the sauce, pour the pork-chop pan juice into the cheese mixture and stir. Let simmer while the pork chops are resting.

7. Put the pork chops on two plates, pour the blue cheese sauce over each other, and serve.

Nutrition:

Calories: 434 Fat: 14.1g Fiber: 11.3g Carbohydrates: 3.1 g Protein: 17.5g

Beef and Vegetable Skillet

Preparation Time: 5 minutes

Cooking Time: 15 minutes

Servings: 2

Ingredients:

- 3 oz spinach, chopped
- 1/2 pound ground beef
- 2 slices of bacon, diced
- 2 oz chopped asparagus

Seasoning:

- 3 tbsp. coconut oil
- 2 tsp. dried thyme
- 2/3 tsp. salt
- 1/2 tsp. ground black pepper

Directions:

1. Take a skillet pan, place it over medium heat, add oil and when hot, add beef and bacon and cook for 5 to 7 minutes until slightly browned.

2. Then add asparagus and spinach, sprinkle with thyme, stir well and cook for 7 to 10 minutes until thoroughly cooked.

3. Season skillet with salt and black pepper and serve.

Nutrition:

Calories: 332 Fat: 18.4g Fiber: 9.4g Carbohydrates: 3.8 g Protein: 14.1g

Beef Taco Salad

Preparation Time: 10 minutes

Cooking Time: 10 minutes

Servings: 2

Ingredients:

- 1-pound ground beef (80/20)
- 1/4 teaspoon pink Himalayan sea salt
- 1/4 teaspoon freshly ground black pepper
- 1/4 cup mayonnaise
- 2 tablespoons sugar-free ketchup
- 2 tablespoons yellow mustard
- 1 tablespoon dill relish
- (8-ounce) bag shredded lettuce
- 1/2 cup sliced red onion
- 1/2 cup chopped ripe tomato
- 1 dill pickle, sliced
- 1/4 cup shredded cheddar cheese

Directions:

1. In a medium sauté pan or skillet, brown the ground beef, stirring, for 7 to 10 minutes. Season with salt and pepper, then drain the meat, if desired. In a small bowl, combine the mayonnaise, ketchup, mustard, and relish.

2. Fill a large bowl with the shredded lettuce. Top with the beef, red onion, tomato, dill pickle, and cheese. Put dressing, serve.

Nutrition:

Calories: 398 Fat: 15.1g Fiber: 12.9g Carbohydrates: 3.1 g Protein: 14.8g

Spinach & Cheese Stuffed Flank Steak Rolls

Servings: 6

Cooking Time: 45 minutes

Ingredients

- 1 ½ lb flank steak
- Salt and black pepper to taste
- 1 cup ricotta cheese, crumbled
- ½ loose cup baby spinach
- 1 jalapeño pepper, chopped
- ¼ cup chopped basil leaves

Directions:

1. Preheat oven to 400° F. Wrap steak in plastic wrap, place on a flat surface, and run a rolling pin over to flatten. Take off the wraps. Sprinkle with half of the ricotta cheese, top with spinach, jalapeño, basil leaves, and remaining cheese.

2. Roll the steak over on the stuffing and secure with toothpicks. Place in a greased baking sheet and cook for 30 minutes, flipping once. Let cool for 3 minutes, slice into pinwheels and serve with sautéed veggies.

Nutrition Info (Per Serving): Cal 490; Net Carbs 2g; Fat 41g; Protein 28g

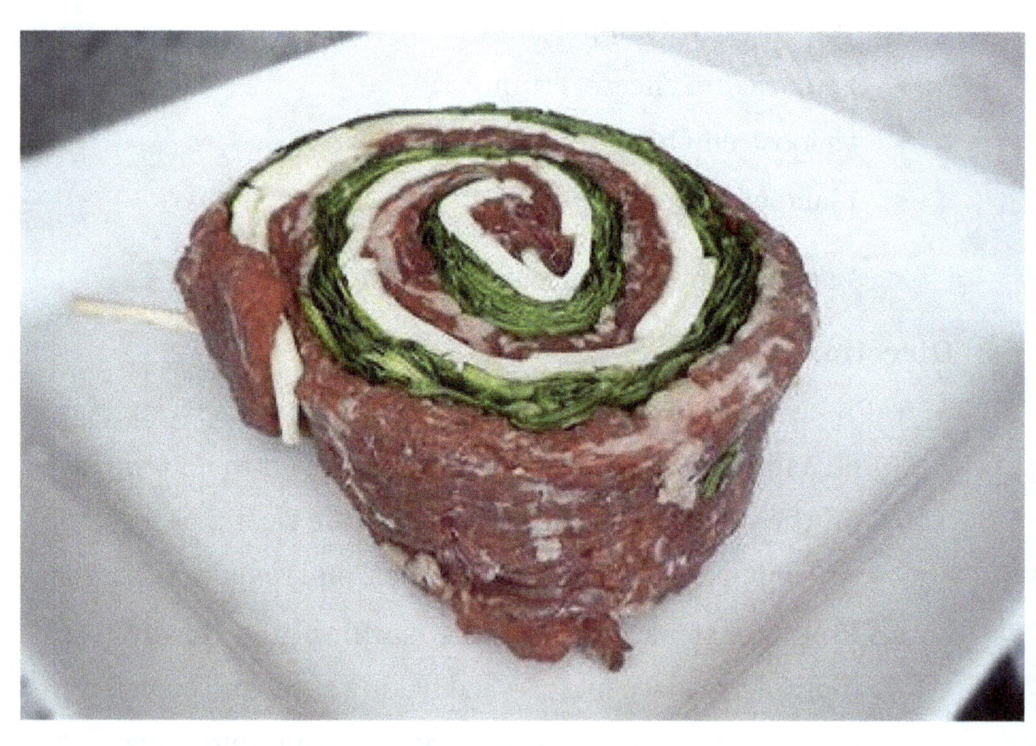

Rolled Lamb Shoulder with Basil & Pine Nuts

Servings: 4

Cooking Time: 1 Hour

Ingredients

- 1 lb rolled lamb shoulder, boneless
- 1 ½ cups basil leaves, chopped
- 5 tbsp pine nuts, chopped
- ½ cup green olives, pitted and chopped
- 3 cloves garlic, minced
- Salt and black pepper to taste

Directions:

1. Preheat the oven to 450° F.

2. In a bowl, combine the basil, pine nuts, olives, and garlic. Season with salt and pepper. Untie the lamb flat onto a chopping board, spread the basil mixture all over, and rub the spices onto the meat.

3. Roll the lamb over the spice mixture and tie it together using 4 strings of butcher's twine. Place the lamb onto a baking dish and cook in the oven for 10 minutes. Reduce the heat to 350°F and continue cooking for 40 minutes. When ready, transfer the meat to a cleaned chopping board; let it rest for 10 minutes before slicing. Serve with roasted root vegetables.

Nutrition Info (Per Serving): Kcal 547, Fat 37.7g, Net Carbs 2.2g, Protein 42.7g

Fantastic Ground Pork with Broccoli

Servings: 4

Cooking Time: 20 minutes

Ingredients

- ½ cup butter
- 5 cups broccoli florets
- 1 lb ground pork
- salt and pepper, to taste
- 1 yellow onion, chopped
- 2 garlic cloves, minced
- ½ teaspoon dried thyme
- 1 tablespoon fresh parsley, chopped
- 2 tablespoons sesame oil

Directions:

1. In a large skillet, heat the sesame oil.

2. Add the ground pork and season with salt, pepper, and thyme. Cook for 7-8 minutes or until it is cooked through. Set aside.

3. In a medium pan, heat up the butter and add the minced garlic; cook for 1 minute.

4. Stir in the broccoli florets, chopped onion and continue cooking for 5-6 minutes. Season with salt, pepper and fresh parsley.

5. Serve the ground pork warm and garnish with the broccoli.

Nutrition Info (Per Serving): 641 Calories; 55.1 Fat; 4g Carbs; 2g Fiber; 32g Protein

POULTRY

63

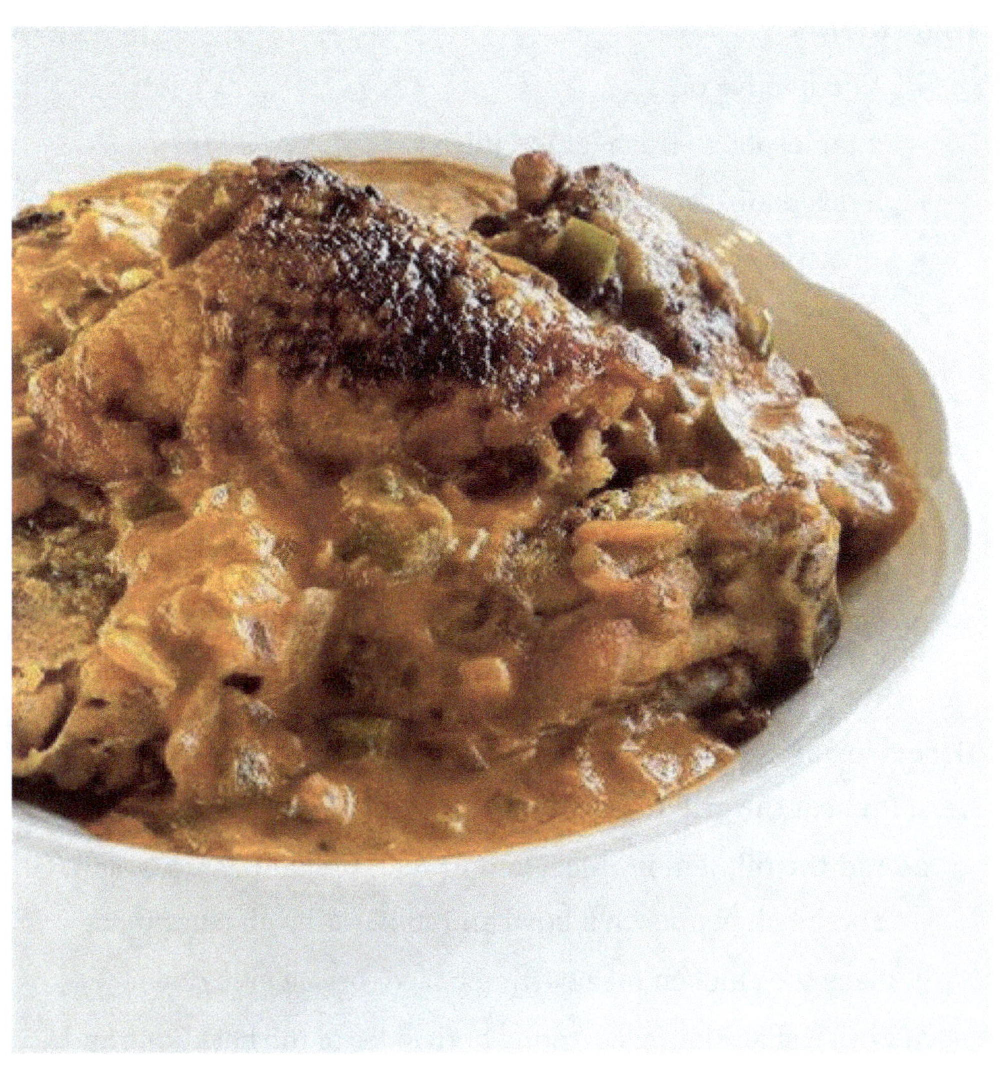

Grilled Whole Chicken

Servings: 6

Cooking Time: 20 minutes

Ingredients

- ¼ cup olive oil
- 2 tablespoons fresh lemon juice
- 2 teaspoons fresh lemon zest, grated finely
- 1 teaspoon dried oregano, crushed
- 2 teaspoons paprika
- 1 teaspoon onion powder
- 1 teaspoon garlic powder
- Salt and ground black pepper, as required
- 1 4-pounds grass-fed whole chicken, neck and giblets removed

Directions:

1. Preheat the grill to medium heat. Grease the grill grate.
2. Add the oil, lemon juice, lemon zest, oregano, spices, salt, and black pepper in a bowl and mix until well combined.
3. Place the chicken on a cutting board, breast side down.
4. With a sharp knife, cut along both sides of the backbone and then remove the backbone.
5. Flip the breast side up and open it like a book.

6. With the palm of your hands, firmly press your breast to flatten.

7. Generously coat the whole chicken with oil mixture.

8. Arrange chicken onto the grill and cook for about 16-20 minutes, flipping once halfway through.

9. Remove from grill and place the chicken onto a cutting board for about 5-10 minutes before carving.

10. Cut into desired size pieces and serve.

Nutrition Info (Per Serving): Calories: 654; Net Carbs: 1g; Carbohydrate: 1.5g; Fiber: 0.5g; Protein: 87.8g; Fat: 31g; Sugar: 0.5g; Sodium: 289mg

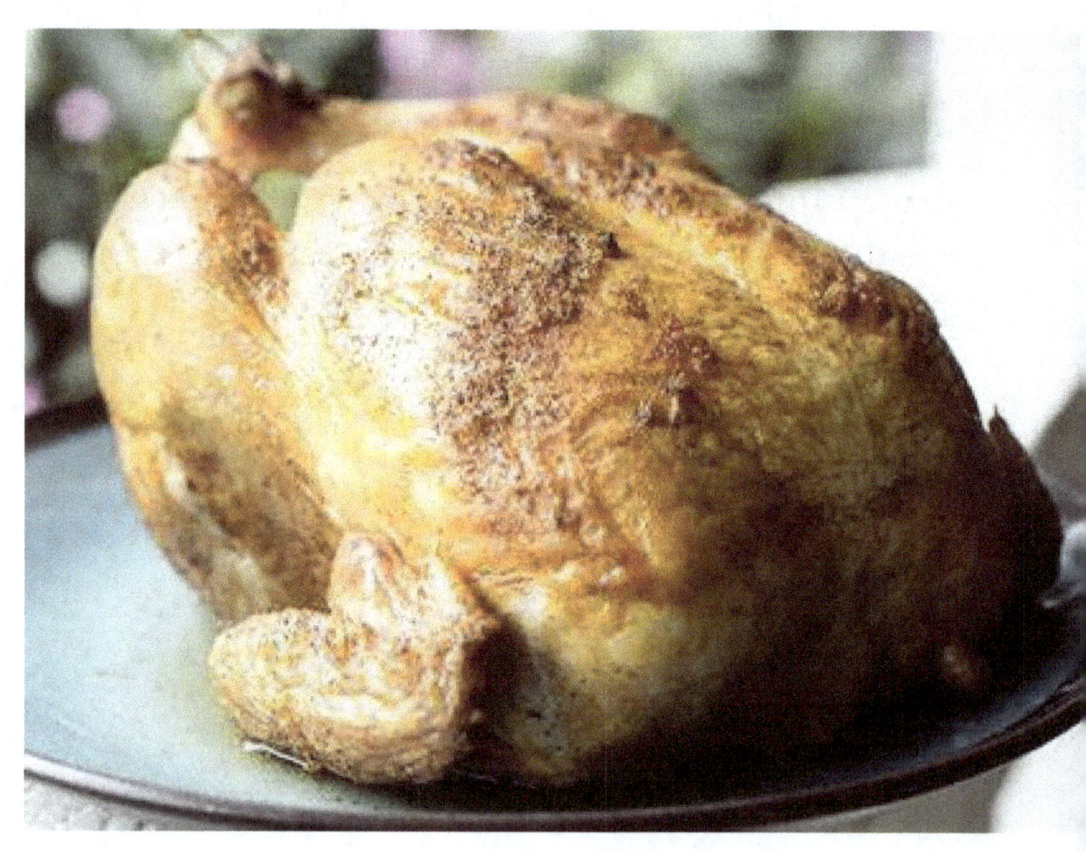

Chicken Breasts with Jarred Pickle Juice

Servings: 4

Cooking Time: 30 minutes

Ingredients

- 2 chicken breasts, cut into strips
- 4 oz chicken crisps, crushed
- 2 cups of coconut oil
- 16 ounces jarred pickle juice
- 2 eggs, whisked

Directions:

1. In a bowl, combine chicken with pickle juice; refrigerate for hours.
2. Place eggs in a bowl and chicken crisps in a separate one.
3. Dip the chicken pieces in the eggs and then in chicken crisps until well coated.
4. Set a pan and warm oil.
5. Fry chicken for 3 minutes per side, remove to paper towels, drain the excess grease, and serve.

Nutrition Info (Per Serving): Cal 387, Net Carbs 2.5g, Fat 16g, Protein 23g

Traditional Hungarian Paprikash

Servings: 5

Cooking Time: 35 minutes

Ingredients

- 2 tablespoons olive oil
- 2 pounds chicken drumsticks
- 1/2 cup leeks, sliced
- 1 bell pepper, deseeded and chopped
- 1 Hungarian wax pepper, chopped
- 3 garlic cloves, chopped
- 1 cup tomato puree
- 4 cups vegetable broth
- Sea salt and freshly ground black pepper, to taste
- 1 tablespoon Hungarian paprika
- 1 bay laurel

Directions:

1. Heat the olive oil in a soup pot over a moderate flame. Once hot, brown the chicken drumsticks for about 7 minutes or until no longer pink; shred the meat and reserve.

2. Then, cook the leeks and peppers in the pan drippings for about 5 minutes or until they have softened.

3. Now, add in the garlic and cook for a minute or so. Add in the tomato puree, vegetable broth, salt, black pepper, Hungarian paprika, and bay laurel.

4. Stir in the reserved chicken and bring to a boil; turn the heat to medium-low, cover, and let it simmer for 22 minutes.

5. Ladle into individual bowls and serve. Enjoy!

Nutrition Info (Per Serving): 358 Calories; 22.2g Fat; 4.4g Carbs; 33.3g Protein; 0.7g Fiber

Bacon Wrapped Chicken with Grilled Asparagus

Servings: 4

Cooking Time: 48 minutes

Ingredients

- 6 chicken breasts
- Pink salt and black pepper to taste
- 8 bacon slices
- 3 tbsp olive oil
- 1 lb asparagus spears
- 3 tbsp olive oil
- 2 tbsp fresh lemon juice
- Manchego cheese for topping

Directions:

1. Preheat the oven to 400° F.

2. Season chicken breasts with salt and black pepper, and wrap bacon slices around each chicken breast. Arrange on a baking sheet that is lined with parchment paper, drizzle with oil and bake for 25-30 minutes until bacon is brown and crispy.

3. Preheat your grill to high heat.

4. Brush the asparagus spears with olive oil and season with salt. Grill for 8-10 minutes, frequently turning until

slightly charred. Remove to a plate and drizzle with lemon juice. Grate over Manchego cheese so that it melts a little on contact with the hot asparagus and forms a cheesy dressing.

Nutrition Info (Per Serving): Kcal 468, Fat 38g, Net Carbs 2g, Protein 26g

FISH

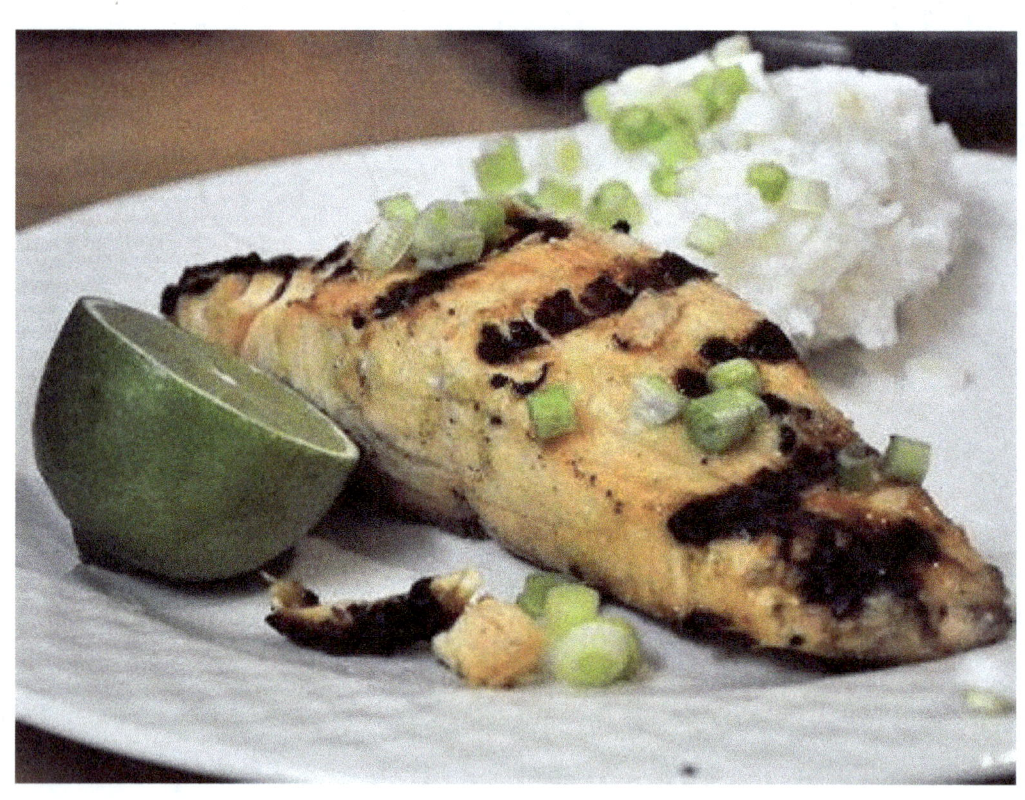

Salmon Cakes

Servings: 3

Cooking Time: 7 minutes

Ingredients

- ¼ cup unsalted butter
- 2 tablespoons fresh rosemary, chopped
- 2 garlic cloves, minced
- 1 pound fresh scallops, side muscles removed
- Salt and ground black pepper, as required

Directions:

1. Melt butter in a skillet, over medium-high heat and sauté the rosemary and garlic for about a minute. Add the scallops and cook for about 2-3 minutes per side or until desired doneness.
2. Season with salt and black pepper and serve hot.

Nutrition Info (Per Serving): Calories: 362; Net Carbs: 1.1g; Carbohydrate: 2.1g; Fiber: 1g; Protein: 40g; Fat: 17.5g; Sugar: 0g; Sodium: 575mg

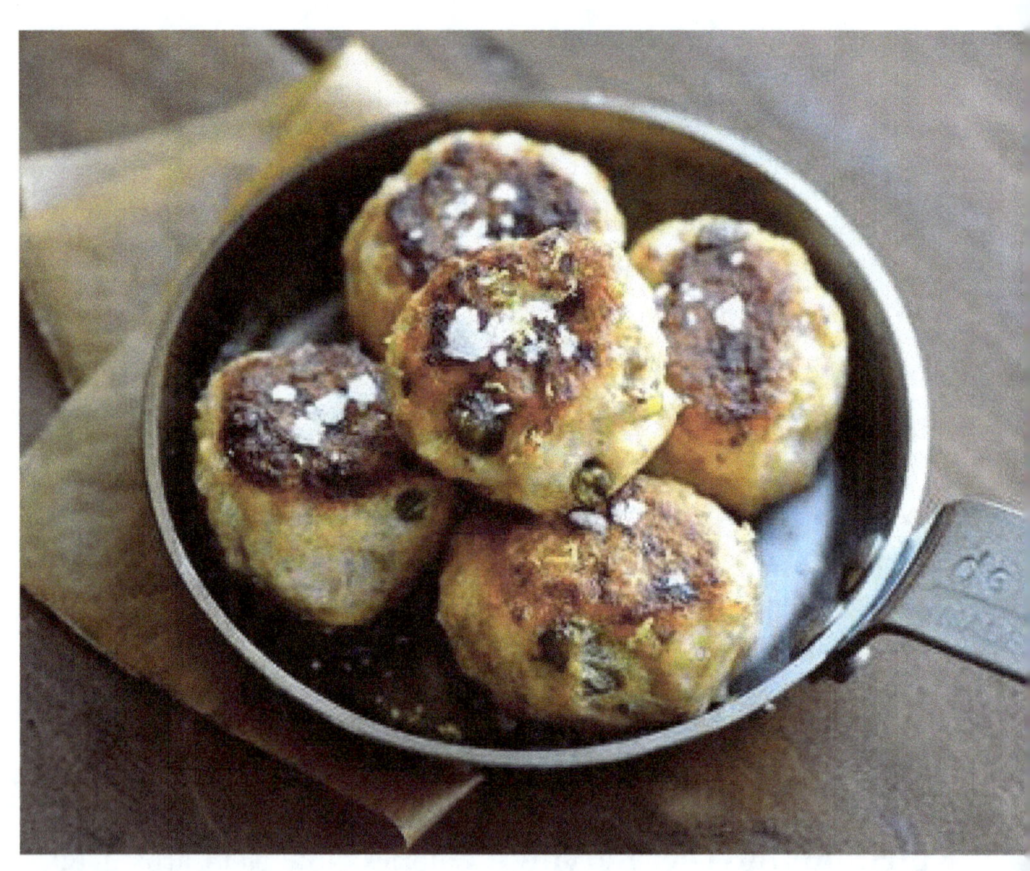

Tasty Sushi Bowl

Servings: 4

Cooking Time: 7 minutes

Ingredients

- 1 ahi tuna steak
- 2 tablespoons coconut oil
- 1 cauliflower head, florets separated
- 2 tablespoons green onions, chopped
- 1 avocado, pitted, peeled and chopped
- 1 cucumber, grated
- 1 nori sheet, torn some cloves sprouts
- For the salad dressing:
- 1 tablespoon sesame oil
- 2 tablespoons coconut aminos
- 1 tablespoon apple cider vinegar
- A pinch of salt
- 1 teaspoon stevia

Directions:

1. Put cauliflower florets in your food processor and blend until you obtain a cauliflower "Rice."

2. Put some water in a pot, add a steamer basket inside, add cauliflower rice, bring to a boil over medium heat, cover, steam for a few minutes, drain and transfer "Rice" to a bowl.

3. Heat up a pan with the coconut oil over medium-high heat, add tuna, cook for 1 minute on each side and transfer to a cutting board.

4. Divide cauliflower rice into bowls, top with nori pieces, cloves sprouts, cucumber, green onions and avocado.

5. In a bowl, mix sesame oil with vinegar, coconut aminos, salt and stevia and whisk well.

6. Drizzle this over cauliflower rice and mixed veggies, top with tuna pieces and serve.

7. Enjoy!

Nutrition Info: calories 300, fat 12, fiber 6, carbs 6, protein 15

Marinated & Grilled Salmon

Servings: 4

Cooking Time: 1 Hour

Ingredients

- 4 5-ounce salmon steaks
- 2 cloves garlic, pressed
- 4 tablespoons olive oil
- 1 tablespoon taco seasoning mix
- 2 tablespoons fresh lemon juice

Directions:

1. Place all of the ingredients in a ceramic dish; cover and let it marinate for 40 minutes in your refrigerator.
2. Place the salmon steaks onto a lightly oiled grill pan; place under the grill for 6 minutes.
3. Turn them over, then cook for a further 5 to 6 minutes, basting with the reserved marinade; remove from the grill.
4. Serve immediately and enjoy!

Nutrition Info (Per Serving): 331 Calories; 21.4g Fat; 2.2g Carbs; 30.4g Protein; 0.4g Fiber

Tuna Egg Wrap

Servings: 2

Cooking Time: 6 minutes

Ingredients

- 2 eggs1 tbsp avocado oil
- 2 oz tuna, packed in water
- 3 tbsp mayonnaise

- Seasoning:
- 1/4 tsp salt
- 1/8 tsp ground black pepper
- ¼ tsp cayenne pepper

Directions:

1. Prepare tuna and for this, place tuna in a medium bowl, add cayenne pepper and mayonnaise and stir until combined.

2. Prepare egg wraps and for this, take a medium bowl, crack eggs in it, add salt and black pepper, and then whisk until blended.

3. Take a frying pan, place it over medium-low heat, add oil and when it melts, pour in half of the egg, spread it evenly into a thin layer by rotating the pan and cook for 2 minutes.

4. Then flip the pan, cook for a minute, and transfer to a plate.

5. Repeat with the remaining egg to make another wrap, divide tuna between wraps, then roll each egg wrap and serve.

Nutrition Info: 321.5 Calories; 28.6 g Fats; 15.3 g Protein; 0.8 g Net Carb; 0.1 g Fiber;

Tasty Shrimp in Creamy Butter Sauce

Servings: 2

Cooking Time: 30 minutes

Ingredients

- ½ oz grated Parmesan cheese
- 1 egg, beaten in a bowl
- ¼ tsp curry powder
- 2 tsp almond flour
- 12 shrimp, shelled
- 3 tbsp coconut oil
- 2 tbsp curry leaves
- 2 tbsp butter
- ½ onion, diced
- ½ cup heavy cream
- ½ ounce cheddar cheese
- Salt and black pepper to taste

Directions:

1. Combine Parmesan, curry powder, and almond flour in a bowl.

2. Melt the coconut oil in a skillet over medium heat.

3. Dip the shrimp in the egg first, and then coat with the dry mixture.

4. Fry until golden and crispy. In another skillet, melt the
   butter.

5. Add onion and cook for 3 minutes. Add in curry leaves and
   cook for 30 seconds.

6. Stir in heavy cream and cheddar cheese and cook until
   thickened.

7. Add the shrimp and coat well. Adjust the seasoning, and
   serve.

Nutrition Info (Per Serving): Cal 560; Net Carbs 4.3g; Fat
56g; Protein 18g

Calamari Salad

Servings: 4

Cooking Time: 4 minutes

Ingredients

- 2 long red chilies, chopped
- 2 small red chilies, chopped
- 2 garlic cloves, minced
- 3 green onions, chopped
- 1 tablespoon balsamic vinegar
- Salt and black pepper to the taste
- Juice from 1 lemon
- 6 pounds calamari hoods, tentacles reserved
- 3.5 ounces olive oil
- 3 ounces rocket for serving

Directions:

1. In a bowl, mix long red chilies with small red chilies, green onions, vinegar, half of the oil, garlic, salt, pepper and lemon juice and stir well.

2. Place calamari and tentacles in a bowl, season with salt and pepper, drizzle the rest of the oil, toss to coat and place on preheated grill over medium-high heat.

3. Cook for 2 minutes on each side and transfer to the chili marinade you've made.

4. Toss to coat and leave aside for 30 minutes.

5. Arrange the rocket on plates, top with calamari and its marinade and serve.

6. Enjoy!

Nutrition Info: calories 200, fat 4, fiber 2, carbs 2, protein 7

Easy Baked Halibut Steaks

Servings: 2

Cooking Time: 20 minutes

Ingredients

- 2 tablespoons olive oil
- 2 halibut steaks
- 1 red bell pepper, sliced
- 1 yellow onion, sliced
- 1 teaspoon garlic, smashed
- 1/2 teaspoon hot paprika
- Sea salt cracked black pepper, to your liking
- 1 dried thyme sprig, leaves crushed

Directions:

1. Start by preheating your oven to 390 degrees F.

2. Then, drizzle olive oil over the halibut steaks. Place the halibut in a baking dish that is previously greased with a nonstick spray.

3. Top with the bell pepper, onion, and garlic. Sprinkle hot paprika, salt, black pepper, and dried thyme over everything.

4. Bake in the preheated oven for 13 to 15 minutes and serve immediately. Enjoy!

Nutrition Info (Per Serving): 502 Calories; 19.1g Fat; 5.7g Total Carbs; 72g Protein; 1g Fiber

VEGETABLES

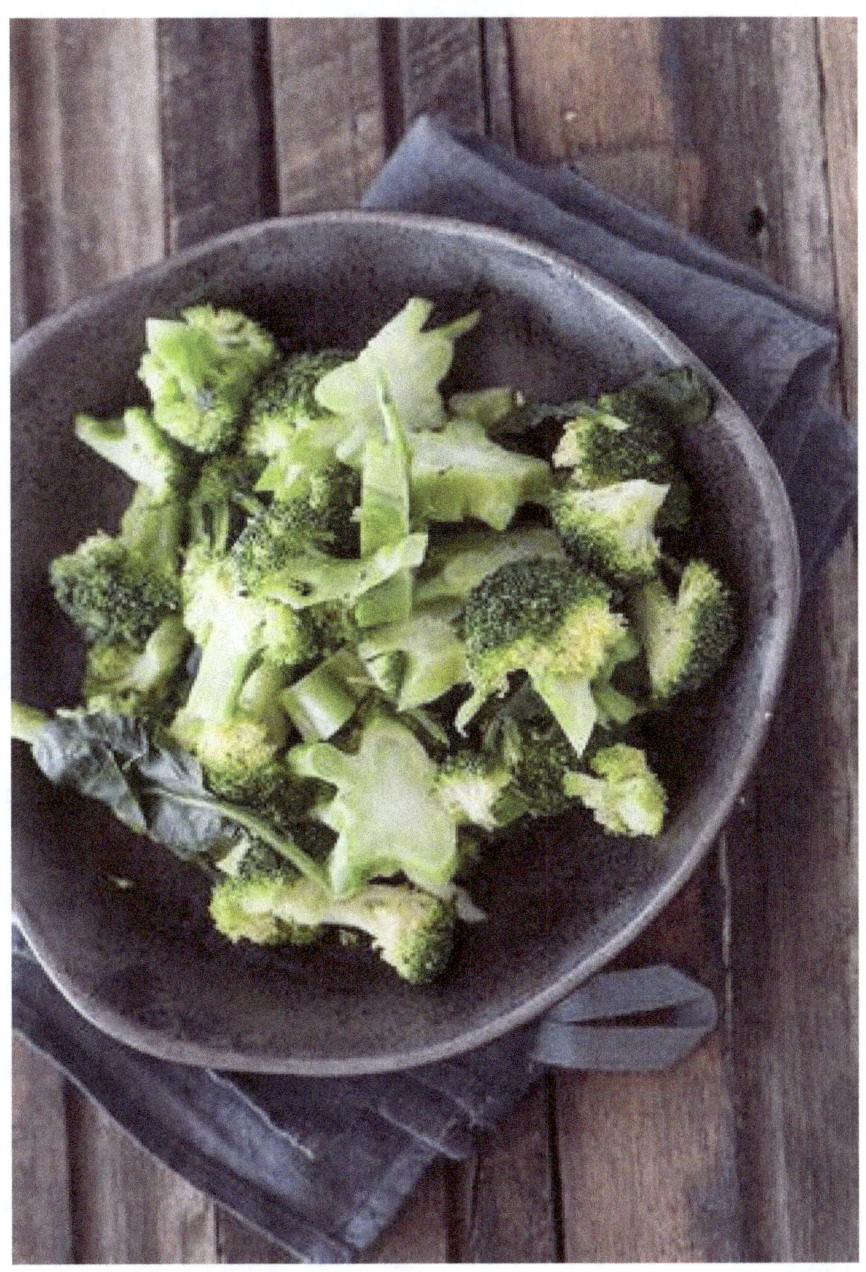

Glazed Carrots

Preparation Time: 19 minutes

Servings: 8

Ingredients:

- 2 pounds baby carrots
- 1/3 cup butter
- 2 tbsp. Erythritol
- 1/2 tsp ground cinnamon
- salt, to taste
- ½ cup of water

Directions:

1. In the pot of Instant Pot, add all ingredients and stir to combine.
2. Secure the lid and place the pressure valve in the "Seal" position.
3. Select "Manual" and cook under "High Pressure" for about 4 minutes.
4. Select the "Cancel" and carefully do a "Natural" release.
5. Remove the lid and serve.

Nutrition Values:

Calories 91, Total Fat 5.9g, Net Carbs 1.56g, Protein 0.8g, Fiber 3.4g

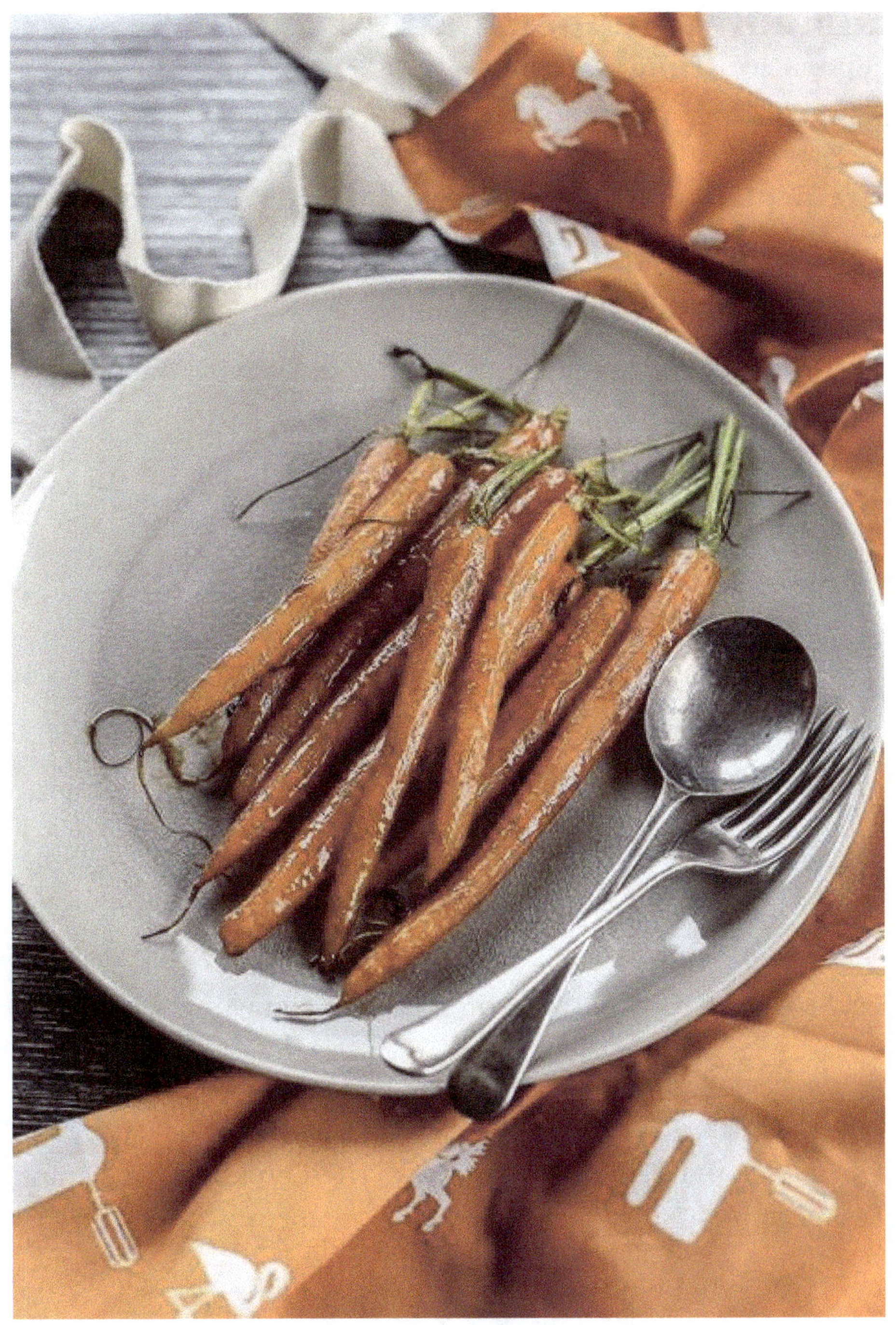

Italian Bell Pepper Platter

Preparation Time: 20 minutes

Servings: 5

Ingredients:

- tbsp. olive oil
- 1 cut into thin strips yellow onion
- 5 seeded and cut into long strips green bell peppers
- very finely chopped medium ripe tomatoes
- chopped garlic cloves
- tbsp. fresh parsley
- Salt and freshly ground black pepper, to taste

Directions:

1. Place the oil in the Instant Pot and select "Sauté." Then add the onion and cook for about 3-4 minutes.
2. Add the bell peppers and garlic clove and cook for about 5 minutes.
3. Select the "Cancel" and stir in the remaining ingredients.
4. Secure the lid and place the pressure valve in the "Seal" position.
5. Select "Manual" and cook under "High Pressure" for about 5-6 minutes.
6. Select the "Cancel" and carefully do a "Quick" release.
7. Remove the lid and serve.

Nutrition Values:

Calories 82, Total Fat 3.2g, Net Carbs 2.7g, Protein 12.4g, Fiber 2.7g

2-Minutes Broccoli

Preparation Time: 12 minutes

Servings: 4

Ingredients:

- cups broccoli florets
- Salt and freshly ground black pepper, to taste

Directions:

1. In the bottom of the Instant Pot, arrange a steamer basket and pour 1 cup of water.
2. Place the broccoli into the steamer basket.
3. Secure the lid and place the pressure valve in the "Seal" position.
4. Select "Manual" and cook under "High Pressure" for about 2 minutes.
5. Select the "Cancel" and carefully do a "Natural" release.
6. Remove the lid and transfer the broccoli to serving plates.
7. Sprinkle with salt and black pepper and serve.

Nutrition Values:

Calories 31, Total Fat 0.3g, Net Carbs 1.52g, Protein 2.6g, Fiber 2.4g

Walnut Roasted Asparagus

Servings: 4

Cooking Time: 20 minutes

Ingredients

- 2 tbsp olive oil
- 1 garlic clove, crushed
- 1 tbsp tamarind sauce
- A handful of walnuts, chopped
- 1 ¼ lb asparagus, trimmed
- 3 tbsp tahini
- 2 tbsp balsamic vinegar
- ½ tbsp chili pepper, chopped

Directions:

1. Preheat oven to 350° F. In a bowl, mix olive oil, garlic, tamarind sauce, and walnuts.

2. Lay asparagus on a baking tray and drizzle tamarind mixture all over.

3. Toss the veggies to coat and roast until tender and charred, minutes.

4. In a bowl, whisk tahini, vinegar, and chili pepper. Plate asparagus, drizzle with dressing, and serve with fried tofu.

Nutrition Info (Per Serving): Cal 359; Net Carbs 8.4g; Fat 32g; Protein 9.6g

Luscious Broccoli Casserole

Preparation Time: 1 hour 4 minutes

Servings: 6

Ingredients:

- 2 tbsp. butter
- 1 chopped small yellow onion
- minced garlic cloves
- 1 cup chopped broccoli florets
- organic eggs
- ¼ cup unsweetened coconut milk
- Salt, to taste
- 1 tsp freshly grated lemon zest
- 1 tbsp. chopped fresh Italian parsley
- 1 tsp chopped fresh thyme
- 1½ cups shredded cheddar cheese

Directions:

1. Grease 1½ quart casserole dish that will fit in an Instant Pot. Keep aside.

2. Place the butter in the Instant Pot and select "Sauté." Then add the onion and garlic and cook for about 7 minutes.

3. Add the broccoli and cook for about 4 minutes.

4. Select the "Cancel" and transfer the broccoli mixture to a large bowl.

5. In a large bowl, add the remaining ingredients except for cheese and beat until well combined.

6. Add broccoli mixture and cheese and stir to combine.

7. Place the mixture into the prepared casserole dish evenly.

8. With the glass lid, cover the casserole dish.

9. In the bottom of the Instant Pot, arrange a steamer trivet and pour 1 cup of water.

10. Place the casserole dish on top of the trivet.

11. Secure the lid and place the pressure valve in the "Seal" position.

12. Select "Manual" and cook under "High Pressure" for about 23 minutes.

13. Select the "Cancel" and carefully do a "Natural" release.

14. Remove the lid and serve warm.

Nutrition Values:

Calories 226, Total Fat 18.6g, Net Carbs 0.68g, Protein 11.7g, Fiber 1g

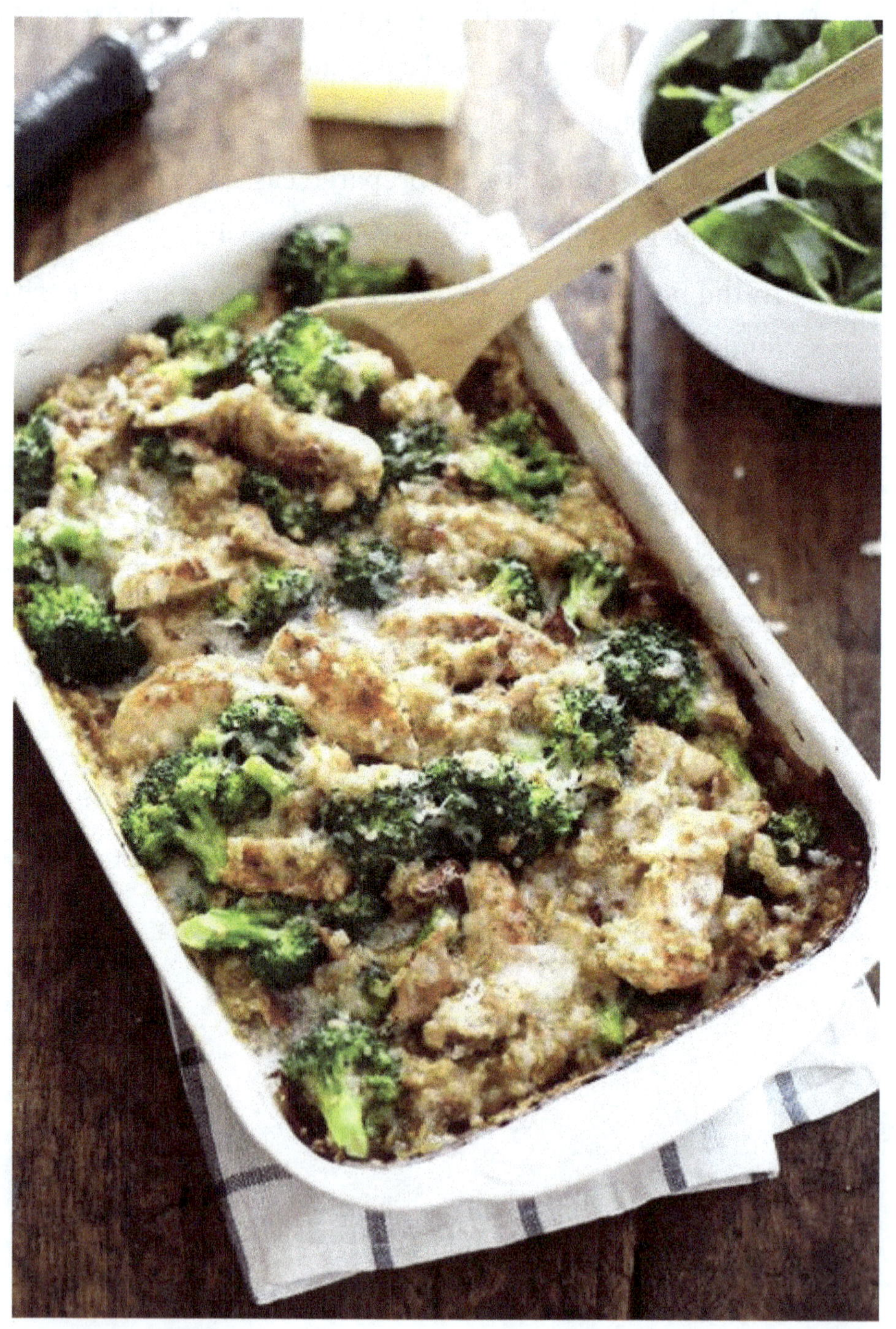

Cabbage Salad

Servings: 6

Cooking Time: 15 minutes

Ingredients

For Salad:

- 4 cups green cabbage, shredded
- ¼ onion, thinly sliced
- 1 teaspoon lime zest, grated freshly
- 3 tablespoons fresh cilantro, chopped

For Dressing:

- ¾ cup mayonnaise
- 2 teaspoons fresh lime juice
- 2 teaspoons chili sauce
- ½ teaspoon Erythritol
- 2 garlic cloves, minced

Directions:

1. For the salad: in a bowl, mix together the cabbage, onion, lime zest and cilantro.
2. For the dressing, add all the ingredients and beat until well combined in another small bowl.
3. Place the dressing over salad and gently toss to coat well.
4. Cover and refrigerate to chill before serving.

Nutrition Info (Per Serving): Calories: 196; Net Carbs: 2.3g; Carbohydrate: 3.6g; Fiber: 1.3g; Protein: 0.7g; Fat: 20.1g; Sugar: 1.7g; Sodium: 231mg

DESSERT

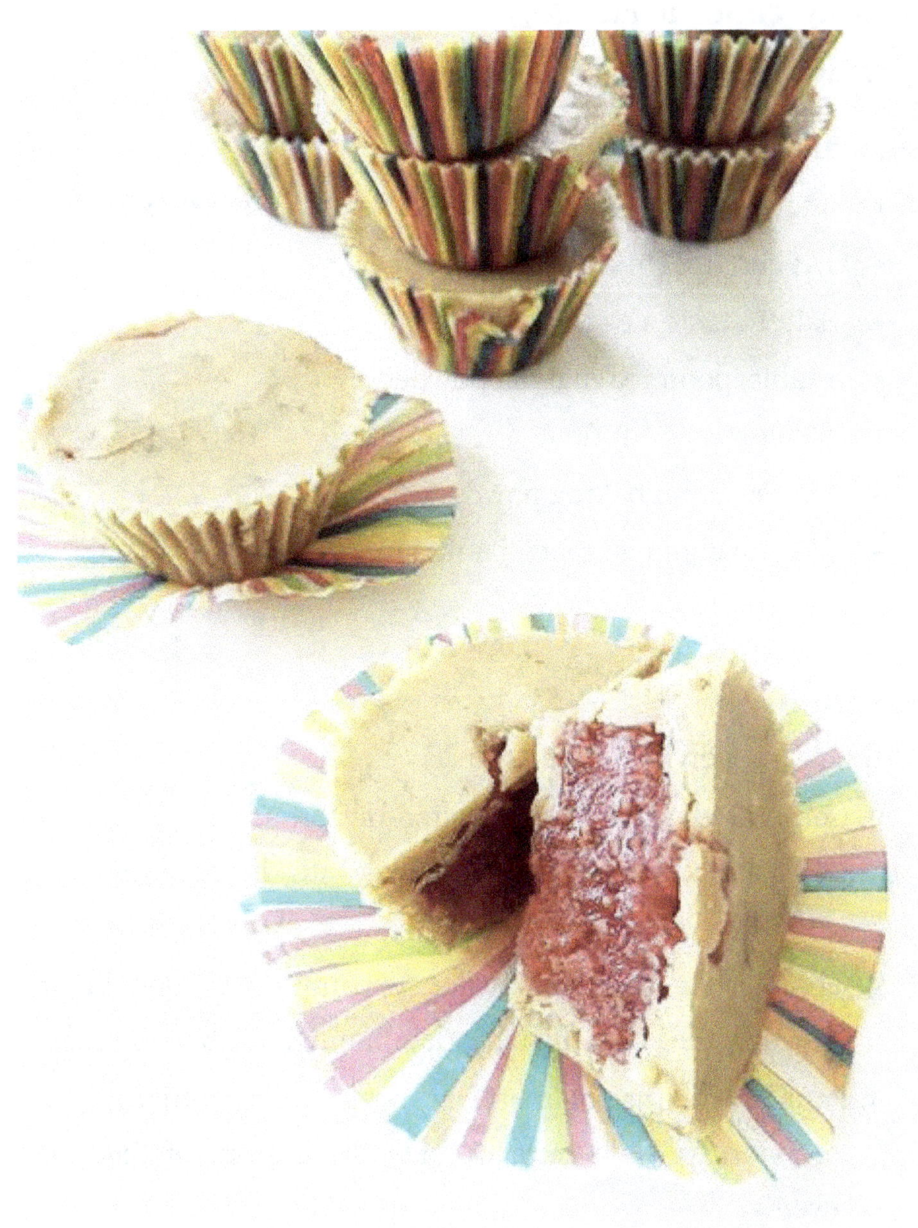

Green Tea and Macadamia Brownies

Preparation Time: 10 minutes

Cooking Time: 20 minutes

Servings: 4

Ingredients:

- 4 tablespoons Swerve confectioners style sweetener
- 1/4 cup unsalted butter, melted
- Salt, to taste 1 egg
- 1 tablespoon tea matcha powder
- 1/4 cup coconut flour
- 1/2 teaspoon baking powder
- 1/2 cup chopped macadamia nuts

Directions:

1. Let the oven heat up to 350° F.
2. Combine the sweetener, melted butter, and salt in a bowl. Stir to mix well. Separate the egg into the bowl, whisk to combine well.
3. Fold in the matcha powder, coconut flour, and baking powder, then add the macadamia nuts. Stir to combine.
4. Pour the mixture on a baking sheet Level the mixture with a spoon to make sure it coats the bottom of the sheet evenly.

5. Bake for 18 minutes or until a sharp knife inserted in the brownies' center comes out clean.

6. Remove the brownies from the oven and slice to serve.

Nutrition:

Calories: 241 Fat: 15.9g Fiber: 6.0g Carbohydrates: 12.1 g Protein: 9.6g

Sesame Cookies

Preparation Time: 15 minutes

Cooking Time: 15 minutes

Servings: 12

Ingredients:

- 1/3 cup monk fruit sweetener, granulated
- 3/4 teaspoon baking powder
- 1 cup almond flour
- 1 egg
- 1 teaspoon toasted sesame oil
- 1/2 cup grass-fed butter, at room temperature
- 1/2 cup sesame seeds

Directions:

1. Let the oven heat up to 350° F.
2. The dry ingredients must be combined in a bowl.
3. The wet ingredients must be mixed in a separate bowl.
4. Pour the wet mixture into the bowl for the dry ingredients. Stir until the mixture has a thick consistency and forms a dough.
5. Put the sesame seeds in a third bowl.
6. Divide and shape the dough into 16 11/2-inch balls, then dunk the balls in the bowl of sesame seeds to coat well.

7. Bash the balls until they are 1/2 inch thick, then put them on a baking sheet lined with parchment paper.

8. Keep a little space between each of them. Baking Time (15 minutes)

9. Remove the cookies from the oven and allow to cool for a few minutes before serving.

Nutrition:

Calories: 174 Fat: 12.4g Fiber: 12.5g Carbohydrates: 8.5 g Protein: 6.8g

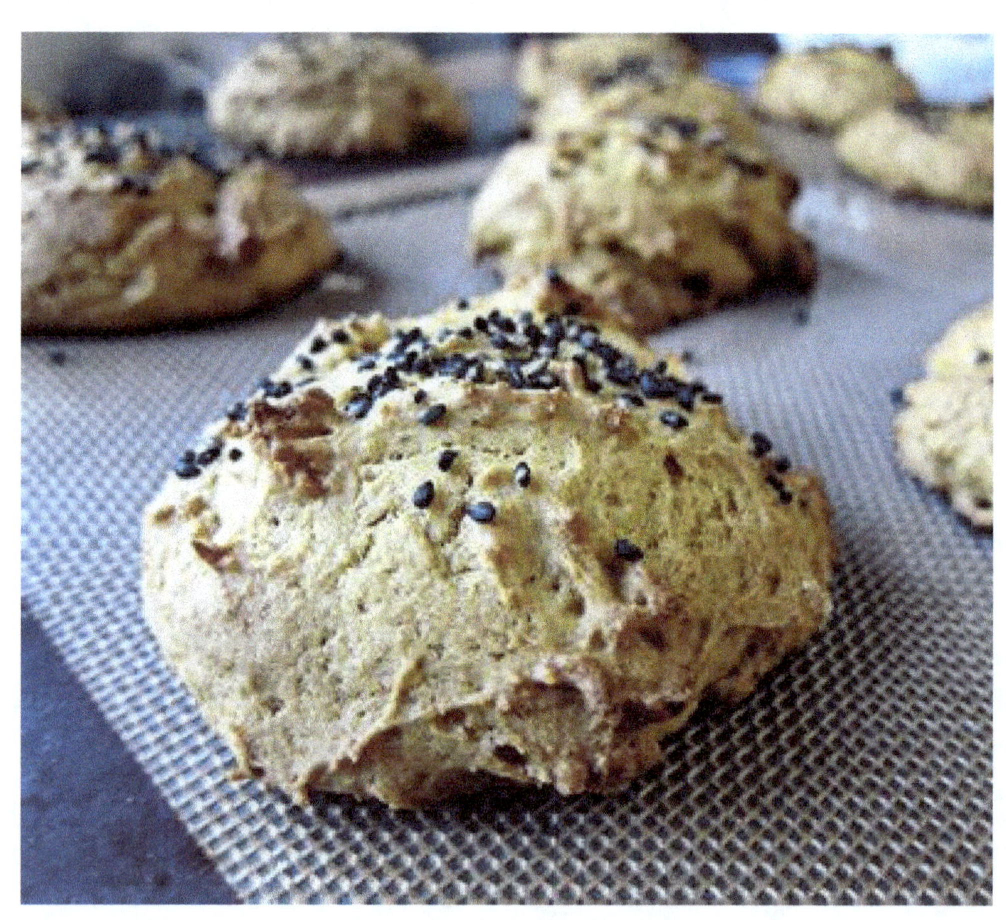

Almond Milk Panna Cotta

Preparation Time: 15 minutes

Cooking Time: 5 minutes

Servings: 4

Ingredients:

- 11/2 C. unsweetened almond milk, divided
- 1 tbsp. unflavored powdered gelatin
- 1 C. unsweetened coconut milk
- 1/3 C. Swerve
- 3 tbsp. cacao powder
- 2 tsp. instant coffee granules
- 6 drops liquid stevia

Directions:

1. In a large bowl, add 1/2 C. of almond milk and sprinkle evenly with gelatin.
2. Set aside until soaked.
3. In a pan, add the remaining almond milk, coconut milk, Swerve, cacao powder, coffee granules, and stevia and bring to a gentle boil, stirring continuously.
4. Remove from the heat.
5. In a blender, add the gelatin mixture and hot milk mixture and pulse until smooth.

6. Transfer the mixture into serving glasses and set aside to cool completely.

7. With plastic wrap, cover each glass and refrigerate for about 3-4 hours before serving.

Nutrition:

Calories: 190 Fat: 8.4g Fiber: 2.5g Carbohydrates: 1.5 g Protein: 1.6g

Lemon Almond Coconut Cake

Preparation Time: 20 minutes

Cooking Time: 40-45 minutes

Servings: 8

Ingredients:

- 250g almond
- 60g desiccated coconut
- Pinch of salt
- 150g natural sugar
- 1 teaspoon vanilla extract zest of
- 1 large lemon
- 3 eggs
- 200g butter, melted
- A handful of almond flakes

Directions:

1. Preheat oven to 180° C.

2. In a medium bowl, take almond, coconut, salt, sugar, vanilla, and lemon zest. Mix in remaining ingredients.

3. Pour in a cake pan. Scatter with almond flakes.

4. Bake for approximately 40-45 minutes until lightly browned and cooked through the middle.

Nutrition:

Calories: 314 Fat: 12.4g Fiber: 6.1g Carbohydrates: 3.1 g Protein: 3.9g

PB& J Cups

Preparation Time: 20 minutes

Cooking Time: 5 minutes

Servings: 4

Ingredients:

- 1/4 cup of water
- 1 teaspoon gelatin
- 3/4 cup of coconut oil
- 3/4 cup raspberries
- 6 to 8 tablespoon Stevia
- 3/4 cup peanut butter

Directions:

1. Line a muffin pan with parchment paper.
2. In a pan, combine the raspberries and water over medium heat. Bring to a boil and then reduce the heat and let the water dry.
3. Mash the berries with a fork. Add in 2 to 4 tablespoons of the powdered sweetener.
4. Add in the gelatin and set aside to cool. Now make a peanut butter mixture.
5. In the pan, put the peanut butter and coconut oil. Cook for 30 to 60 seconds, until melted.
6. Also, add in 2 to 4 tablespoons of the powdered sweetener.

7. Put half of the peanut butter mixture in a muffin pan and put in the freezer to firm up for about 15 minutes.

8. Divide the raspberry mixture among the muffin cups and top with the remaining peanut butter mixture. Refrigerate until firm.

Nutrition:

Calories: 191 Fat: 6.1g Fiber: 2.2g Carbohydrates: 1.8 g Protein: 3.1g

Mini Blueberry Cheesecakes

Preparation Time: 35 minutes

Cooking Time: 10 minutes

Servings: 6

Ingredients:

For crust:

- 1 cup almond flour
- 1 tbsp. sweetener
- 2 tbsp. coconut oil
- 1/4 tsp. vanilla extract
- Pinch of salt

For cheesecake

- 8 oz cream cheese
- 1/2 cup sweetener
- 1 cup sour cream
- 1 tsp. vanilla extract

Blueberry topping

- 1 cup fresh blueberries
- 2 tbsp. water
- 1/2 tbsp. lemon juice
- 1/4 tsp. xanthan gum

Directions:

1. For the crust: In a bowl, mix almond flour, sweetener, coconut oil, vanilla extract, and salt, stir well and make the dough.

2. Take muffin cups and place dough evenly in cups. Bake them for 8 minutes in a preheated oven at 325C until golden brown.

3. Cheesecake filling: in a bowl, have cream cheese and beat with an electric beater, now add sweetener and beat until turn fluffy.

4. In a bowl, mix sour cream and cheese cream mixture with vanilla extract and mix well.

5. Now fill the crust with cheesecake filling and cool for an hour.

6. Blueberry sauce: in a pan, put blueberries, water, and lemon juice and cook on medium flame, now turn flam low and add xanthan gum and stir for 2 to 3 minutes.

Nutrition:

Calories: 276 Fat: 10.4g Fiber: 2.3g Carbohydrates: 1.8 g Protein: 3.8g